# Radiology Words and Phrases

## A Quick-Reference Guide

### Second Edition

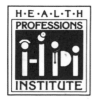

Health Professions Institute • Modesto, California • 1990

# Radiology Words and Phrases:
## A Quick-Reference Guide
## Second Edition

*Published by:*

Health Professions Institute
P. O. Box 801
Modesto, California 95353
Telephone (209) 524-4351

Sally C. Pitman, Editor & Publisher

*Printed by:*
Parks Printing & Lithograph
Modesto, California

ISBN 0-934385-18-1

Last digit is the print number: 9 8 7 6 5 4 3

# Acknowledgments

This reference book was produced by the staff and associates of Health Professions Institute: Susan M. Turley, CMT, RN, BSN, Curriculum Coordinator, Baltimore; Linda C. Campbell, CMT, Educational Coordinator, Modesto; Vera Pyle, CMT, Consulting Editor, San Francisco; and John H. Dirckx, M.D., Medical Consultant, Dayton, Ohio.

In addition, we wish to thank individuals who have supplied word lists and other resource materials: Shirley Bell, CMT, Walkersville, Maryland; Catherine Gilliam, CMT, Houston, Texas; Nancy Isaacs, Columbia, Maryland; Susan Pierce, CMT, Herndon, Virginia; and Linda Vourlogianes, Petaluma, California.

Our warmest gratitude to all.

Sally C. Pitman, CMT, MA
Editor & Publisher

# Preface

The primary source for *Radiology Words and Phrases: A Quick-Reference Guide,* 2nd edition, is *The SUM Program Radiology Transcription Unit* (1987) and *A SUM Plus Exercise in Radiology Transcription* (1988). These educational materials are part of The SUM (Systems Unit Method) Program for Training Medical Transcriptionists.

This second edition contains more than 10,000 medical words and phrases drawn from the latest textbooks and medical journals in radiology and its subspecialties as well as hundreds of actual transcripts of radiology dictation on bones and soft tissues, contrast studies and interventional radiology, nuclear medicine, ultrasonography, mammography, computerized tomography scans, and magnetic resonance imaging reports.

The radiology words and phrases in this book are listed alphabetically and are extensively cross-referenced. An eponymic title may be located alphabetically as well as under the term that it modifies. For example, *Omnipaque contrast medium* may be found under both *Omnipaque* and the main entry *contrast medium.* For simplicity and consistency, eponyms are not presented in the possessive form ('s), although they are frequently used as possessives in medical dictation and in the literature. To minimize unnecessary duplications, many subentries are combined under one main entry. The main entry *fracture* includes all fractures which are also found alphabetically throughout the book. Main entries with multiple subentries include:

| | | |
|---|---|---|
| angiogram | duct | notch |
| angle | film | obstruction |
| aorta | fold | pattern |
| arteriogram | fracture | pneumonia |
| bone | gallbladder | polyp |
| calcification | gastritis | radioisotope |
| calculus | heart | scan |
| catheter | hernia | sign |
| contrast medium | image, imaging | sinus |
| defect | infiltrate | study |
| deformity | joint | syndrome |
| density | kidney | ulcer |
| disease | lesion | ultrasound |
| dislocation | line | units of measure |
| diverticulum | node | view |

# Radiology Words and Phrases

# A, a

A-mode
A ring, esophageal
A-scan (ultrasound)
Abbokinase
abdomen
  acute
  postlymphangiography
  postsurgical
abdominal aorta
abdominal aortic aneurysm
abdominal carcinosis
abdominal pregnancy
abduction
aberrant
abnormal tracer accumulation
abnormality
  definitive
  fetal
  focal
  perfusion
aboral direction
abruption
abruption of placenta
abruptio placentae
abscess
  appendiceal
  Brodie
  Paget
absorber
absorptiometry
  double photon (DPA)
  single photon (SPA)
absorption, bony

absorption coefficient
abut, abutting
acanthopelvis
ACAT (automated computerized
  axial tomography)
accelerated peristalsis
accelerator, linear
accentuation of markings
accessory bone
accessory center of ossification
accessory sinus
accumulation, abnormal tracer
ace of spades sign on angiogram
acetabular bone
acetabular cup
acetabular fossa
acetabular notch
acetabular prosthesis
acetabular roof
acetabulum, deep-shelled
acetazolamide
achalasia
Achilles bursa
Achilles tendon
AC (acromioclavicular) joint
ACG (apexcardiogram)
achondroplasia
achondroplastic
acinus (pl. acini)
acoprosis
acoprous
acoustical shadowing
acoustic impedance

acoustic interface
acoustic shadowing
acquisition time
acromegaly
acromial angle
acromial bone
acromiale os secondarium
acromioclavicular (AC) joint
acromiocoracoid ligament
acromiohumeral
ACS angioplasty Y connector
ACS guide wire
ACS Indeflator
ACS LIMA guide
ACS RX coronary dilatation
  catheter
ACS SULP II balloon
actinomycosis
activation analysis
activity, cardiac
Acuson computed sonography
Acuson linear array (5 MHz)
Acuson transvaginal sonography
acute abdominal series
acute renal failure (ARF)
adactyly
Addison point
adductor canal
adductor hiatus
adductor tubercle
adenocarcinoma
adenoma, bronchial
adenomatosis
adenomatous hyperplasia
adenopathy
  bronchopulmonary
  celiac
  cervical
  iliac
  inguinal
  mesenteric
  periaortic

adenopathy *(cont.)*
  perihilar
  perivertebral
  prevertebral
  subcarinal
adhesions, pleural
adhesive, Surgical Simplex P
  (radiopaque bone cement)
adiabatic demagnetization
adiabatic fast passage
adipose ligament
adipose tissue
aditus pelvis
adnexa, adnexal (not adnexae)
adrenal gland
adrenal scintiscanning
ADR ultrasound
adult respiratory distress syndrome
  (ARDS)
adynamic ileus
aerate, aerated
aeration
aerophagia
afferent loop
afferent view
affix, affixed
age, gestational
agenesis of lung
agenesis, renal
agenetic fracture
aggregated follicles
aglutition
AICA (anterior inferior
  communicating artery)
air
    free
    intramural colonic
    intraperitoneal
air bronchogram
air contrast barium enema
air contrast study
air cystogram

air-fluid level
air inflation
air sac
air-space disease
air trapping, localized
airway
Akerlund deformity
ala cerebelli
ala cinerea
ala ilii
ala lobuli centralis
ala magna
ala, nasal (pl. alae)
ala nasi
ala parva
ala pontis
ala sacralis
ala vomeris
alar bone
Albers-Schönberg disease
Albers-Schönberg marble bones
Albert disease
Alderson average-man random
   phantom
alignment
   anatomic
   poor
   rotational
alignment of fracture fragments
alignment, vertebral
alimentary canal
Allis sign
Alouette amputation
Aloka color Doppler imaging
Aloka linear scanner
Aloka sector scanner
Aloka ultrasound diagnostic
   equipment
alpha particle
alveolar bone
alveolar consolidative process
alveolar edema

alveolar infiltrate
alveolus (pl. alveoli)
Alzheimer disease
ambon
amenorrhea
Amipaque contrast medium
amniography
amniotic fluid
amniotic sac
amorphous
Amplatz dilator
Amplatz needle
amplifier, linear
ampulla of Vater
ampulla recti
amputation
   Alouette
   Beclard
   Callander
   Carden
   Chopart
   Hey
   Le Fort
   Pirogoff
   Syme
   Teale
   Vladimiroff-Mikulicz
amyloid disease
anal atresia
anal sphincter
analog to digital converter
analysis
   activation
   digital frequency
anamnesis
anastomosis
   Billroth II
   Braun
   colocolic
   ileorectal
   pyeloileocutaneous
   Roux-en-Y

anastomosis *(cont.)*
   transureteroureteral
   ureteroileocutaneous
   ureteroureteral
anatomic alignment
anatomic neck of humerus
anatomic position
anatomic snuffbox
anatomy
anconeal fossa (also anconal fossa)
ancyroid cavity (also ankyroid)
android pelvis
anechoic area
anemia
   aplastic
   Biermer
   iron deficiency
   sickle cell
anencephaly
anesthesia, anesthetic
aneurysm
   abdominal aortic
   berry
   calcified wall of
   dissecting
   innominate
   mural
   popliteal
   thoracoabdominal aortic
aneurysmal dilatation of abdominal
   aorta
Anger camera
angiocardiography
Angiocath
Angio-Conray contrast medium
angiogram, -graphy
   biplane orthogonal
   Brown-Dodge method for
   cardiac
   carotid
   celiac
   cerebral

angiogram *(cont.)*
   cine-
   contrast
   coronary
   digital subtraction (DSA)
   ECG-synchronized digital sub-
      traction
   equilibrium radionuclide
   first-pass nuclide rest and
      exercise
   first-pass radionuclide
   fluorescein
   gated blood pool
   gated nuclear
   gated radionuclide
   left ventricular
   pancreatic
   post angioplasty
   PTCA coronary
   pulmonary
   pulmonary artery wedge
   radionuclide (RNA)
   renal
   rest and exercise gated nuclear
   selective coronary cine-
   single plane
   sitting-up view
   transvenous digital subtraction
   ventricular
angiogram suite
Angiografin contrast medium
angiographic gap at site of injury
angiographic variceal embolization
angiographically
angiography (see *angiogram*)
angioma
angioplasty, balloon
angiopneumography
angioscope, Optiscope flexible
   fiberoptic
Angioskop-D
Angiovist contrast medium

angle
  acromial
  antegonial
  Bauman
  blunted costophrenic
  blunting of costophrenic
  blunting of costovertebral
  Boehler (Böhler)
  cardiophrenic
  carrying
  cerebellopontile (CPA)
  cerebellopontine (CPA)
  costal
  costophrenic (CP)
  costosternal
  costovertebral (CVA)
  flip
  gonial (of the mandible)
  Louis
  Ludwig
  Mikulicz
  obliterated costophrenic
  pontine
  radiocarpal
  Ranke
  sternal
  sternoclavicular
  urethrovesical
  valgus carrying
  vertebrophrenic
  vesicourethral
  xiphoid
angle of inclination of urethra
angstrom
angular frequency
angular momentum
angularis sulcus
angulated fracture
angulus costae
angulus sterni
anhaustral colonic gas pattern
anion

anisotropic 3-D or volume study
ankle mortise
ankle mortise fracture
ankylosing spondylitis
ankylosis of joint
ankyroid cavity (also ancyroid)
annular
annulus ovalis
annulus umbilicalis
anomaly
  aortic arch
  cardiac
  congenital
  congenital cardiac
antecubital fossa
antecubital space
anteflexion
antegonial angle
antegonial notch
antegrade blood flow
antegrade fashion
antegrade ureteral stent
anterior arch of the atlas
anterior compartment syndrome
anterior inferior communicating
  artery (AICA)
anterior inferior iliac spine
anterior inferior spine of ilium
anterior maxillary spine
anterior rectopexy
anterior superior iliac spine (ASIS)
anterior superior spine of ilium
anterior tibial artery
anterofundal placenta
anterolisthesis
anteroposterior (AP)
  (also anterior-posterior)
anteversion
anthracosilicosis
anthropoid pelvis
anticoincidence circuit
antifibrin antibody imaging

antral edema
antral gastritis
antrum cardiacum
antrum, gastric
antrum pyloricum
anvil bone
aorta
  abdominal
  aneurysmal widening of
  ascending
  bifurcation of
  calcified
  coarctation of
  descending
  ectasia of abdominal
  ectasia of thoracic
  elongated
  elongation of
  elongation of thoracic
  overriding
  retroesophageal
  stenosis of
  thoracic
  tortuous
  wide tortuous
  widening of
aortic aneurysm
aortic angiography
aortic arch angiography
aortic bifurcation
aortic calcification
aortic coarctation
aortic configuration of cardiac
  shadow
aortic dissection
aortic flush pigtail catheter
aortic flush straight catheter
aortic insufficiency
aortic knob
aortic notch
aortic root
aortic septal defect

aortic stenosis
  calcific
  subvalvular
  supravalvular
aortic valve
  calcified
  ectatic
  gradient
  nodules of
  opening of
  prolapse of
  stenosed
  thickened
aortic valve leaflet prolapse
aortic valve opening
aortic valve, thickened
aortic window
aorticopulmonary fenestration
aorticopulmonary window
aortocaval fistula
aortofemoral arterial runoff
aortofemoral arteriogram
aortofemoral bypass graft
aortofemoral runoff
aortogram
  abdominal
  antegrade
  arch
  contrast
  digital subtraction
  digital subtraction supravalvular
  flush
  postangioplasty
  retrograde
  retrograde femoral
  retrograde transaxillary
  retrograde translumbar
  supravalvular
  thoracic arch
  translumbar
aortography
  balloon occlusive

aortography *(cont.)*
  biplanar
  counter-current
  retrograde transfemoral
  selective visceral
aortoiliac
aortovelography, transcutaneous
  (TAV)
AP (anteroposterior or anterior-
  posterior) film, projection, view
AP supine portable view
apex (pl. apices)
apexcardiogram (ACG)
aphagia
apical cap
apical granuloma
apical impulse
apical view
apically directed chest tube
apices (pl. of apex)
aplasia
aponeurosis
  bicipital
  epicranial
apophyseal fracture
apophyseal joint
apophysis of Rau
apophysitis tibialis adolescentium
apoplexy
  Broadbent
  cerebellar
  pulmonary
appendage
  cecal
  vermicular
appendiceal abscess
appendices or appendixes (pl.)
appendicolith
appendix
  ensiform
  filiform
  retrocecal

appendix *(cont.)*
  vermiform
  xiphoid
appendix caeci
appendixes or appendices (pl.)
appendix vermiformis
apple core lesion
apposition, close
approximate
approximation
aproctia
aqueduct, cerebral
aqueduct of Sylvius
arachnodactyly
Aran-Duchenne disease
arbor alveolaris
arborescent
arcade of collaterals
Arcelin view
arch
  aortic
  hemal
  neural
  Riolan
  subpubic
  zygomatic
arch of atlas
architecture
  hepatic
  lobular
archocele
arcuate eminence
arcuate ligament
ARDS (adult respiratory distress
  syndrome)
area
  anechoic
  Haeckerman
  hyperechoic
  hypoechoic
  mitral
  rarefied
  suprapubic

areola
areolar
argentaffinoma of bronchus
argentaffinoma of GI tract
Arnold convolution
array
   convex
   high-density
   linear
   phased
   symmetrical phased
array processor
arrest, epiphyseal
arterial graft
arterial occlusion
arterial runoff
arteriogram, -graphy
   aorta and runoff
   arch
   biplane pelvic
   biplane quantitative coronary
   brachial
   brachiocephalic
   carotid
   celiac
   cerebral
   cine-
   coronary
   femoral
   four-vessel
   hepatic
   infrahepatic
   intraoperative
   Judkins technique for coronary
   left coronary cine-
   longitudinal
   lumbar
   mesenteric
   percutaneous
   percutaneous femoral
   peripheral
   pruned-tree

arteriogram *(cont.)*
   pulmonary
   pulmonary artery
   renal
   retrograde
   runoff
   selective
   selective coronary
   Sones selective coronary
   subclavian
   superior mesenteric
   vertebral
   visceral
   wedge
arteriosclerosis, peripheral
arteriosclerotic plaque
arteriosclerotic thoracoabdominal
   aortic aneurysm
arteriosus, ductus
arteriovenous aneurysm
arteriovenous fistula
artery
   abdominal aorta
   anterior inferior communicating
     (AICA)
   axillary
   brachial
   cannulated
   carotid
   celiac
   common carotid
   common femoral
   common iliac
   coronary
   external carotid
   external iliac
   iliac
   innominate
   inferior mesenteric
   internal carotid
   internal iliac gluteal
   mesenteric

artery *(cont.)*
  popliteal
  posterior tibial
  profunda femoris
  renal
  subclavian
  superficial femoral
  superior mesenteric
  ulnar
  vertebral
arthritides (pl. of arthritis)
arthritis
  degenerative
  hypertrophic
  post-traumatic
  presby-
  rheumatoid
arthritis deformans
arthrogram, -graphy
  Brostrom-Gordon
  double contrast
  Gordon-Brostrom
  single contrast
arthrogryposis multiplex congenita
arthropathy, neurogenic
arthrosclerosis
arthrosis deformans
arthrotomography of shoulder,
  double contrast
articular cartilage
articular facet
articular fracture
articular fragment
articular gout
articular process
articular surface
articulation
  acromioclavicular
  atlantoaxial
  metacarpophalangeal (MP)
  sacroiliac
  talonavicular

articulatio talocruralis
articulatio talonavicularis
artifact, artifactual
arytenoid cartilage
asbestos
asbestosis
ascending aorta
ascending colon
Aschoff node
ascites, ascitic
aseptic necrosis
ASIS (anterior superior iliac spine)
aspect
  medial
  posterolateral
aspiration pneumonia
assay, radioisotope clearance
assessment, real-time
asthenic
asthma, potter's
astragalar bone
astragalocalcanean
astragalocrural
astragaloscaphoid bone
astragalotibial
astragalus, fracture of
astroblastoma
astrocytoma
asymmetrical narrowing of artery
asymptomatic
atelectasis
  basilar
  bibasilar
  platelike
  platter-like
  segmental
  subsegmental bibasilar
atelectatic
atherosclerosis, atherosclerotic
Atkin epiphyseal fracture
ATL Mark 600 real-time sector
  scanner

ATL real-time NeuroSectOR
    scanner
atlantoaxial articulation
atlantoaxial joint
atlantoaxial separation
atlanto-occipital fusion; junction
atlanto-odontoid
atlas (C1; first cervical vertebra)
atonic esophagus
atony, atonic
atresia
    anal
    biliary
    congenital biliary
    congenital laryngeal
    duodenal
    esophageal
    extrahepatic biliary (EBA)
    intestinal
    intrahepatic (IHA)
    laryngeal
    prepyloric
atrial appendage
atriography, contrast left
atrioseptal defect
atrioventricular septum
atrium, respiratory
atrophic fracture
atrophied
atrophy
    cerebral
    disuse
    Duchenne muscular
    Hoffmann
    muscle
    quadriceps
    Sudeck

attenuated lumen
attenuation, valve
atypical
auditory meatus
Auerbach plexus
auricle, auricular
auricular fissure
automated computerized axial
    tomography (ACAT)
autoradiograph
avascular necrosis
avulse, avulsed
avulsion chip fracture
avulsion fracture
avulsion fracture of spinous process
avulsion of epiphysis
avulsion, traumatic
axial compression fracture
axial compression injury of spine
axial dimension
axial images, multi-echo
axial loading of spine
axial plane
axial scan
axial section
axilla, axillae
axillary adenopathy
axillary node
axis (C2; second cervical vertebra)
axis
    basibregmatic
    basicranial
    celiac
Ayerza syndrome
azygos lobe
azygos vein

# B, b

B-mode
B ring, esophageal
B-scan (ultrasound)
Babinski reflex
Babinski sign
background subtraction technique
backscattering
backwash ileitis
baker leg (genu valgum)
bald gastric fundus
ball-and-socket joint
balloon angioplasty
balloon catheter, Orion
balloon French shaft
balloon occlusive aortography
balloon-tipped catheter
balloon tuboplasty
ball-valve obstruction
Bamberger-Marie disease
band
    His
    Lane
band of density
Banti disease
Barclay niche
barber pole sign
Bard bioptic gun
Bardex tube
Bardinet ligament
Baricon contrast medium
barium
    residual
    retained
barium column, head of
barium, double tracking of
barium enema (BE)
    air contrast
    double contrast
    full column

barium enema through colostomy
barium esophagram
barium injection (through
    colostomy)
barium meal
barium suspension
barium sulfate contrast medium
barium suspension, oral
barium swallow
Barkow ligament
Baro-CAT contrast medium
Baroflave contrast medium
Barosperse contrast medium
barrel chest
barrel-shaped chest
Barrett esophagus
barrier, blood-brain (BBB)
Barton fracture
basal, basally
basal ganglia
basal neck fracture
base
    lung
    skull
base of thumb
baseline of bulb
baseline, Reid
baseline tenting (BLT)
basibregmatic axis
basicranial axis
basilar atelectasis
basilar region
basilar neck fracture
basilar pneumonitis
basilar sulcus
basioccipital bone
basion
basis cerebri
basis cordis

bathycardia
bathygastria
bat-wing formation
Baudelocque diameter
Bauhin valve
Bauman angle
bayonet leg
bayonet position of fracture
BB (metallic foreign body)
BBB (blood-brain barrier)
BE (barium enema)
beaded appearance of fibro-
    muscular dysplasia
beaking of head of talus
beam dosimetry
    adjacent field x-ray
    four-field x-ray
    large-field x-ray
    single x-ray
beam, fan
beam linear accelerator, high-
    energy bent
bear claw ulcer
beaten silver appearance
Beau disease; syndrome
Beauvais disease
Beck gastrostomy
Beclard amputation
Beclard hernia
becquerel (Bq)
bed
    gallbladder
    hepatic
    liver
    portal vascular
    ulcer
Bekhterev disease
Bell-Dally dislocation
bending fracture
benign
benignity
Bennett fracture at base
    of metacarpal

Bentson guide wire
Bentson introducer
Berman angiographic catheter
berry aneurysm
Bertel position
beryllium granulomatosis
beta decay
beta particle
betatron
bezoar
bibasally
bibasilar atelectasis
biceps femoris muscle
Bichat canal
bicipital aponeurosis
bicipital rib
bicipital tuberosity
biconcave
bicondylar fracture
bicornuate uterus
bicuspid
Biermer anemia
bifid
bifurcation, hepatic duct
bifurcation of aorta
bifurcation of common bile duct
bi-ischial diameter
bilateral, bilaterally
bilateral facet dislocation of
    cervical spine
Bilbao-Dotter catheter
Bilbao-Dotter tube
bile duct
bile duct proliferation
bile duct scan
bile flow
bilharziasis
biliary atresia
biliary duct
biliary dyskinesia
biliary mud
biliary obstruction

biliary passages
biliary radicle
biliary sludge
biliary stent
biliary structures
biliary tract
biliary tree
Biligrafin contrast medium
Bilivist contrast medium
Billroth II type anastomosis
bilocular stomach
Bilopaque contrast medium
bimalleolar ankle fracture
binge, bingeing (binging)
biological half-life
biological hazards
biometry, longitudinal ultrasonic
biopsy
bioptic gun, Bard
biparietal bossing
biparietal diameter (BPD)
biparietal suture
bipartite patella
biplanar aortography
biplane sector probe
bird-beak configuration or
    narrowing
bird-beak taper at esophagogastric
    junction
bispinous diameter
bite block
bituberous diameter
bivalve, bivalved
bladder, dome of urinary
bladder floor
bleb
blennothorax
blind catheter
blindgut
blind intestine
blind pouch
blink mode

blister of bone
Bloch equation
blood
    epidural
    heparinized
    intraventricular
    parenchymal
    sensitized
    subdural
blood-brain barrier (BBB)
blood flow, antegrade
blood flow study
blood pool, vascular
Blount disease
blow-in fracture
blow-out fracture
BLT (baseline tenting)
blue rubber-bleb nevus syndrome
blue toe syndrome
Blumenbach clivus
blunted costophrenic angle
blunting of costophrenic angle
blunting of posterior sulci
Bochdalek, foramen of
Bochdalek hernia
body
    asteroid
    coccygeal
    esophageal
    foreign
    Gamna-Gandy
    pineal
    scapular
    vermiform
    vertebral
body of scapula
body of stomach
body section radiography
Boeck sarcoid
Boehler (Böhler) angle
Boerhaave syndrome
boggy synovitis

Böhler (Boehler) angle
Boltzmann distribution factor
bolus injection
bombardment
bone
  accessory
  acetabular
  acromial
  alar
  Albers-Schönberg marble
  alveolar
  anvil
  astragalar
  astragalus
  astragalocalcanean
  astragalocrural
  astragaloscaphoid
  astragalotibial
  basilar
  basioccipital
  Bethesda
  breast
  bregmatic
  brittle
  bundle
  calcaneal
  calcaneus
  calf
  cancellated
  cancellous
  capitate
  carpal
  cartilage
  chalky
  chevron (V-shaped)
  coccygeal
  coccyx
  collar
  compact
  continuity of
  cortical
  costal

bone *(cont.)*
  crest of iliac
  cribriform
  crushed
  cuboid
  cuneiform
  dense structure of
  depression of nasal
  diastasis of cranial
  eburnated
  endochondral
  ethmoid
  femoral
  fibula, fibular
  flank (ilium)
  flat
  fracture running length of
  fragmental
  freeze-dried
  frontal
  funny
  greater multangular
  hamate
  heel
  heterotopic
  hip
  humeral
  hyoid
  iliac
  iliac cancellous
  incomplete fracture of
  incus
  infected
  innominate
  interparietal
  intrachondrial
  irregular
  ischial
  ivory
  jaw
  knuckle
  lacrimal

bone *(cont.)*
  lamellar
  lamellated
  lenticular (of hand)
  lesser multangular
  lingual
  long
  long axis of
  lunate
  luxated
  malar
  malleolus, malleolar
  marble
  mastoid
  mature
  maxillary
  membrane
  metacarpal
  metatarsal
  mortise
  multangular
  navicular
  nonlamellated
  occipital
  os calcis
  osteonal
  osteoporotic
  pagetoid
  parietal
  pelvic
  petrous
  Pirie
  pisiform
  porous
  post-traumatic atrophy of
  primitive
  proliferation of
  prominence of
  raw
  refractured
  replacement
  rider's

bone *(cont.)*
  rudimentary
  sacral
  scaphoid
  scapular
  semilunar
  sesamoid
  short
  sphenoid
  splintered
  spoke
  spongy
  stirrup
  subchondral
  substitution
  supernumerary
  suprainterparietal
  supraoccipital
  sutural
  talus
  tarsal
  temporal
  thigh
  tibia
  trabecular
  trapezium
  trapezoid of Henle
  trapezoid of Lyser
  triangular
  tubular
  turbinate
  tympanic
  ulnar
  unciform
  vomer
  whettle
  woven
  xiphoid
  zygomatic
bone absorption
bone age, by Greulich and Pyle
bone age ratio

bone atrophy
bone block
bone cement, Surgical Simplex P
  radiopaque
bone chip
bone debris
bone demineralization
bone density, increased
bone deposits, endochondral
bone destruction, localized
bone destructive process
bone ends
bone erosion
bone formation
  new
  sparsity of
bone-forming sarcoma
bone fracture
bone fragment
bone graft incorporation
bone imaging
bone infarct
bone island
bonelet
bone marrow
bone mass, loss of
bone maturation, normal
bone metastases, occult
bone mineralization
bone or joint pathology
bone plug
bone remodeling
bone resorption
bone resurfacing
bone scan
  isotope
  TSPP rectilinear
bone shaft
bone spicule
bone spur
bone stock, poor
bone substance

bone survey
bone window
bony abnormality
bony ankylosis
bony apposition
bony architecture
bony bridging
bony callus formation
bony change
bony deformity
bony deposit
bony destruction, area of
bony disruption
bony enlargement
bony excrescence
bony exostosis
bony fragment
bony fusion
bony healing
bony island
bony landmark
bony necrosis and destruction
bony osteophytes
bony pelvis
bony prominence
bony protuberance
bony reabsorption, subchondral
bony resorption
bony sclerosis
bony skeleton
bony spicule
bony spur, spurring
bony stability
bony structure
bony structures, demineralized
bony thorax
bony union, solid
boot-shaped heart
boot-top fracture
borborygmus (pl. borborygmi)
borderline
boss

bosselated, bosselation
bossing, biparietal
Bosworth procedure
Bosworth screw
Botallo duct
Botallo foramen
Botallo ligament
both bone forearm fracture
Bouchard disease
boutonniere deformity of finger
bowel
   aganglionic
   apple-peel
   dead
   dilated loops of
   distal small
   fluid-filled loop of
   infarcted
   intussuscepted
   irritable
   ischemic
   large
   multiple loops of small
   proximal small
   small
   strangulated
bowel contents
bowel continuity
bowel fills and evacuates
   satisfactorily
bowel follow-through, small
   (SBFT)
bowel gas pattern
bowel gas, superimposed
bowel loop
bowel lumen
bowel motion
bowel obstruction, complete
bowel pattern
bowel prep (preparation)
bowel series, small
bowel shadows, superimposition of

bowel syndrome
   irritable
   spastic
bowel wall
bowleg (genu varum)
bowler hat sign
Bowman capsule
boxer's fracture of metacarpal
BPD (biparietal diameter)
Bq (becquerel)
brachial
brachiocephalic artery
brachiocubital
brachiocyllosis
brachiocyrtosis
brachium
brachycephaly
brachydactyly
brachytherapy, remote afterloading
   (RAB)
Bragg curve
brain scan
brain stem
branched calculus
branches of the vein
branch, muscular
Braun anastomosis
Braun tumor
breast
   atrophic
   chicken
   pendulous
   pigeon
   tail of
breast bone or breastbone
breast mass lesion, with poorly
   defined margins
breast shadow
breech presentation
bregmatic bone
Breuerton view of hand
bridge of meniscus

bridging
  bony
  ventral
bridging osteophytes
Brinton disease
Bristow procedure for dislocated
  shoulder
brittle bone
broad-based
Broadbent apoplexy
Brodie abscess
Brodie bursa
Brodie disease
Brodie knee
Brodie ligament
bronchi (pl. of bronchus)
bronchial adenoma
bronchial stenosis
bronchial tree
bronchiectasis
  capillary
  cylindrical
  cystic
  follicular
  saccular
bronchiole
bronchiolitis
bronchitis
bronchoalveolar
bronchocele
bronchogenic
bronchogram, -graphy
bronchopneumonia
bronchopulmonary atelectasis
bronchopulmonary segment
bronchospasm
bronchovascular markings,
  crowding of
bronchovesicular
bronchus, main stem (pl. bronchi)
brow presentation
Bruck disease

BRW (Brown-Roberts-Wells) CT
  stereotaxic guide
bubble ventriculography
bucardia
bucket-handle fracture
Buck extension
Bucky view
Budlinger-Ludlof-Laewen disease
buffalo hump
bulb
  baseline of
  duodenal
bulge, disk
bulging
bulla, bullae
bullous emphysema
bumper fracture
bunamiodyl contrast medium
bundle
  Kent-His
  Pick
bundle bone
bundle of His
bunion
bunk bed fracture
Burdach, column of
bursa
  Brodie
  Fleischmann
  Monro
  plantar
  popliteal
  prepatellar
  suprapatellar
bursa anserina
bursa omentalis
bursa tendinis calcanei
bursitis
  olecranon
  radiohumeral
burst fracture
bursting fracture

Busquet disease
butterfly fracture
butterfly fracture fragment
butterfly-type glioma
button
   patellar
   Murphy

buttonhole fracture
button of duodenum
bypass graft

# C, c

C1–C7 (seven cervical vertebrae)
C–arm fluoroscopy
C–loop of duodenum
C sign
cachexia
   lymphatic
   thyroid
caecum (cecum)
Caffey disease
calcaneal bone
calcaneal fracture
calcaneal spur
calcaneitis
calcaneoapophysitis
calcaneoastragaloid
calcaneocavus
calcaneoclavicular ligament
calcaneocuboid joint
calcaneonavicular coalition
calcaneotibial fusion
calcaneovalgocavus
calcaneus, calcaneal
calcar
calcar femorale
calcar pedis
calcareous
calcarine fissure
calcific
calcification
   aortic
   cerebral

calcification *(cont.)*
   coarse vascular
   conglomerate
   coronary artery
   curvilinear
   dystopic
   eggshell-like
   fine
   gyriform
   intervertebral cartilage
   intervertebral disk
   intracranial
   irregular
   ligamentous
   medial collateral ligament
     of knee
   Mönckeberg
   mottled
   multiple
   Pellegrini-Stieda
   periarticular
   periductal
   pineal gland
   premature
   secondary
   soft tissue
   stippled
   valvular
calcification of artery
calcification of cartilage
calcification of choroid plexus

calcification of costal cartilages, premature
calcification of intervertebral cartilage
calcified aortic valve
calcified cartilage
calcified density
calcified free body
calcified granuloma
calcified hilar node
calcified lesion
calcified lymph node
calcified mass
calcified node
calcified pericardium
calcified pineal gland
calcified plaque
calcified thyroid adenoma
calcified valve
calcified wall of aneurysm
calcifying hematoma
calcium deposition
calculus (pl. calculi)
    alternating
    biliary
    branched
    cholesterol
    gallbladder
    gastric
    hepatic
    impacted
    intestinal
    laminated
    lucent
    mulberry
    nephritic
    nonopaque
    opaque
    pancreatic
    prostatic
    radiopaque
    renal

calculus *(cont.)*
    staghorn
    stomach
    ureteral
    urinary tract
Caldani ligament
Caldwell occipitofrontal view
caliber of lumen
calibrator
caliceal system
caliectasis
calix, caliceal (or calyx, calyceal)
callosal dysgenesis
callosum, corpus
callus (n.), callous (adj.)
callus formation (not *callous*)
callus, fracture
calvarial
calvarium (pl. calvaria)
Calvé-Perthes disease
calyx, calyceal (or calix, caliceal)
camera, gamma
Camurati-Engelmann disease
canal
    alimentary
    Bichat
    haversian
    medullary
    Nuck
    semicircular
    spinal
cancellated bone
cancellous bone
cancellous screw
cancellus (n.); cancellous (adj.)
Cannon-Boehm point
Cannon point
Cannon ring
Cannon segmentation
cannula, cannulation
cap
    duodenal

cap *(cont.)*
  knee
  phrygian
capillary fracture
capital epiphysis (CE) angle
capitate bone
capitellum
capitulum costae
capitulum fibulae
capitulum humeri
capitulum mandibulae
capitulum radii
capitulum ulnae
capsular ligament rupture
capsule
  Glisson
  internal
  joint
capsuloperiosteal envelope
caput medusae
carcinoid
carcinoma, scirrhous
carcinomatosis, lymphangitic
carcinosis, abdominal
Carden amputation
cardia
  gastric
  patulous
cardia of stomach
cardiac activity
cardiac antrum
cardiac compensation
cardiac decompensation
cardiac dilatation
cardiac effusion
cardiac failure
cardiac gating
cardiac impression on liver
cardiac monitor
cardiac notch
cardiac scan
cardiac silhouette

cardiac stomach
cardiac tamponade
cardioangiography
cardioangioscope, Sumida
cardioesophageal (CE) junction
Cardiografin contrast medium
cardiogram, -graphy
  apexcardiogram (ACG)
  esophageal
  precordial
  ultrasonic (UCG)
  vector
cardiomegaly, borderline
cardiophrenic angle
cardiopulmonary
cardiospasm
cardiothoracic (CT) ratio
cardiovascular
Carey-Coons stent
carina fornicis
carina of trachea
Caroli disease
carotid angiography
carotid artery
carotid vein
carpal bone
  central
  first
  fourth
  great
  intermediate
  radial
  second
  third
  ulnar
carpal navicular
carpal tunnel syndrome
carpometacarpal articulation; joint
Carr-Purcell-Meiboom-Gill sequence
carrying angle
Carswell grapes
cartilage bone

cartilage, softening and swelling of
cartilaginous foreign bodies in
   joint cavity
cartwheel fracture
cascade stomach
caseous pneumonia
Castaneda internal-external drain
catarrh, gastric
catarrhal pneumonia
cathartic
catheter
   angiographic
   angiographic balloon occlusion
   angiopigtail
   aortic flush pigtail
   aortic flush straight
   aortogram
   balloon
   balloon-dilating
   balloon-tipped angiographic
   bat-wing
   Berman angiographic
   Bilbao-Dotter
   biliary balloon
   biliary drainage
   blind
   cannulation
   cholangiography
   Cobra
   Cobra 2
   Cope loop
   coudé
   Councill
   dilating
   drainage
   ERCP (endoscopic retrograde
     cholangiopancreatography)
   externally draining
   femoral aortic flush
   femoral visceral renal curve
   Fogarty balloon biliary
   French 5 angiographic

catheter *(cont.)*
   Grollman pigtail
   Groshong
   Gruentzig (or Grüntzig)
   H-1-H (headhunter)
   headhunter visceral angiographic
   Hickman
   Hieshima coaxial
   H/S (hysterosalpingography)
   hydrostatic balloon
   Infuse-a-port
   internal-external drainage
   intra-arterial
   intrahepatic biliary drainage
   introducer
   JB1
   JB3
   Jelco
   jugular
   Lehman ventriculography
   Malecot
   Mallinckrodt angiographic
   Mani
   Medi-Tech
   midstream aortogram
   Millar pigtail angiographic
   Mitsubishi angioscopic
   mushroom
   NIH left ventriculography
   Nycore angiography
   Orion balloon
   percutaneous transhepatic pigtail
   pigtail
   portal
   PTBD (percutaneous trans-
     hepatic biliary drainage)
   Ring
   Ring-McLean
   Rosch
   Royal Flush angiographic flush
   Seldinger
   short-arm Grollman

catheter *(cont.)*
    Simmons 1; 2; 3
    sidewinder
    Softip arteriography
    subclavian
    Swan-Ganz
    Tennis Racquet angiographic
    Torcon NB selective angiographic
    umbilical
    ventriculography
catheter advanced under fluoro-
    scopic control
catheter exchanged over a guide
    wire
catheterization
CAT (computerized axial
    tomography)
CAT scan
    enhanced
    nonenhanced
catheter tip
caudad, caudal
cauda equina
caudate lobe
cauliflower-shaped filling defect
caval
cavernous
cavitation
Cavitron ultrasonic aspirator
    (CUSA)
cavity
    abdominal
    ancyroid (also ankyroid)
    sigmoid
cavogram, -graphy
cavum Vergae
cc (cubic centimeter)
CDH (congenital dysplasia of hip)
CE (capital epiphysis) angle
CE (cardioesophageal) junction
cecal appendage
cecal sphincter

cecal volvulus
cecostomy
cecum (caecum) mobile
celiac
celiac axis
celiac ganglia
celiac plexus
celiectasia
celioma
celitis
cella lateralis
cella media
cement, radiopaque bone
centigray (cGy)
centimeter (cm)
central canal
centriciput
centrum commune
cephalad
cephalic presentation of fetus
cephalometry
cephalopelvic disproportion (CPD)
cephalopelvimetry
cerclage
cerebellar apoplexy
cerebellopontile angle (CPA)
cerebellopontine angle (CPA)
cerebellum, cerebellar
cerebral angiography
cerebral aqueduct
cerebral atrophy
cerebral brain flow
cerebral hemisphere
cerebral infundibulum
cerebral white matter
cerebri, falx
cerebrospinal fluid (CSF)
cerebrovascular accident (CVA)
Cerenkov radiation
cervical CT (computed tomography)
cervical esophagus
cervical myelogram

cervical outlet
cervical rib
cervical spinal cord
cervical spine
cervical triangle
cervicothoracolumbosacral
cervicotrochanteric fracture
cervix (adj. cervical)
cervix uteri
cesarean section
CGR biplane angiographic system
cGy (centigray)
chain, obturator nodal
chain of lakes deformity
chain of lakes filling defect
chain of lakes sign
chalasia
chalky bone
chamber
   ionization
   Wilson cloud
Chamberlain-Towne view
chance fracture
change
   cystic
   degenerative
   fibrotic
   lytic
channel
   deep venous
   pyloric
characteristic, echo
Charcot foot
Charcot joint
Charcot-Marie-Tooth disease
Chausse view
cheek bone
chemical shift
chemotherapy
chest
   barrel
   flail

chest (cont.)
   funnel
   phthinoid (flat)
chest tube, apically directed
Chester disease
chevron bone (V-shaped)
CHF (congestive heart failure)
Chiari II malformation
Chiba needle
chicken breast
Chilaiditi syndrome
chip fracture
chiropractic films
chisel fracture
choana cerebri
choanal
Cholangiocath
cholangiocatheter
   cystic duct
   saline-filled
cholangiofibromatosis
cholangiogram, -graphy
   balloon
   Chiba percutaneous
   common duct
   contrast selective
   cystic duct
   endoscopic retrograde (ERC)
   fine-needle percutaneous
   fine-needle transhepatic
   intraoperative
   intravenous (IVC)
   operative
   percutaneous transhepatic
   serial
   T-tube (TTC)
   thin-needle percutaneous
   transhepatic (THC)
cholangiopancreatography, endoscopic retrograde (ERCP)
cholangioscope, peroral
cholangioscopy, intraductal

Cholebrine contrast medium
cholecystectasia
cholecystectomized
cholecystectomy
cholecystitis
cholecystocholangiogram, -graphy
cholecystoduodenostomy
cholecystogram, oral
cholecystokinin
cholecystolithiasis
cholecystopathy
cholecystoptosis
cholecystoscopy, percutaneous
    transhepatic
choledochal
choledochoduodenostomy
choledochoenterostomy
choledochofiberoscopy
choledochojejunostomy
choledocholith
choledochotomy
cholelith
cholelithiasis
cholelithotomy
cholescintigram, -graphy
cholescintography radionuclide test
cholesteatoma
cholesterosis
Cholografin meglumine contrast
    medium
chololith
chondral fragment
chondrocalcinosis
chondrodystrophy
chondroma
chondromalacia of patella
chondrosternal
Chopart amputation
Chopart ankle dislocation
chordae tendineae
choroid plexus

Christmas tree appearance of
    pancreas
chronic obstructive pulmonary
    disease (COPD)
chronic synovitis of knee
Ci (curie)
cicatricial contraction
cicatrizing enteritis
cineangiogram, -graphy
    aortic root
    biplane
    coronary
    left ventricular (LV)
    radionuclide
    selective coronary
    Sones technique for
cine-esophagogram
cine-esophagoscopy
cinefluorography
cinefluoroscopy
Cine Memory with Color Flow
    Doppler imaging
cineventriculogram, -graphy
circle of Willis
Circon video camera
circuit
    anticoincidence
    coincidence
circulation, collateral
circumference
    abdominal
    head
    thigh
circumferential fracture
circumferentially
circumscribed infiltrate
cirrhosis, Laennec
cirrhotic
cistern, prepontine
cisternogram, -graphy
    CT
    metrizamide CT (MCTC)

cisternogram *(cont.)*
　oxygen
Clado point
clavicle, clavicular
clavicular notch
clawfoot deformity
clawhand deformity
clawtoe deformity
clay shoveler's fracture
clearance of contrast material
clearance, radioactive xenon
cleavage fracture
cleft foot
cleft lip
cleidocranial dysostosis
clinical correlation
clip
　metallic
　skin
　surgical
clivus, Blumenbach
close-up
closed-break fracture
closed dislocation
closed fracture
clot-filled lumen
cloverleaf deformity
cloverleaf nail
cloverleaf skull
Cloward back fusion
clubbing of fingers and toes
clubfoot
cm (centimeter)
C/N (contrast-to-noise) ratio
coalescence
coarctation of aorta
coarse vascular calcification
coating
coaxial catheter, Hieshima
coaxial sheath cut-biopsy needle
cobblestoned appearance of
　pancreas

Cobra 2 catheter
coccidioidomycosis
coccygeal body
coccygeal bone
coccygeopubic diameter
coccyx, coccygeal
codivilla extension
coefficient, absorption
coeur en sabot
coherent scattering
coil
　crossed
　Golay
　gradient
　Helmholtz
　receiver
　RF (radiofrequency)
　shim
　solenoid
　surface
coiled spring appearance of intus-
　suscepted bowel
coincidence circuit
coin-shaped lesion
cold nodule
colectomy
colitis
　myxomembranous
　ulcerative
colitis polyposa　　　　　•
colitis ulcerosa gravis
collar bone
collar-button appearance in colon
collateral circulation
collateral edema
collateral eminence
collateralization
collaterals, parenchymal
collateral vessel
collecting system
collection of contrast material
Colles fracture

colliculus
collimated
collimation
collimator
  parallel-hole
  pinhole
collision, inelastic
colloid shift on liver-spleen scan
colocolic anastomosis
colocutaneous fistula
colon
  ascending
  descending
  distal
  diverticulum of
  elongation of
  emptying of
  giant
  iliac
  inflammation of
  irritable
  lead-pipe
  left
  loops of redundant
  midsigmoid
  obstruction of
  pelvic
  proximal
  redundancy of
  right
  saccular
  sigmoid
  spastic
  transverse
colonic diverticulum
colonic pit
colonic polyp
colonoscopy
coloptosis
colorectal cancer
Color Flow Doppler real-time
  2-D blood flow imaging

colostomy
colovesical fistula
colpocele
colpoptosis
column
  contrast
  Lissauer
column of Burdach
column of contrast medium
column of Morgagni
columnar
columning of dye
comminuted bursting fracture
comminuted intra-articular fracture
comminuted teardrop fracture
commissure of tectum
common bile duct
common duct cholangiogram
common duct stone
common femoral artery
common iliac artery
compact bone
compartment, medial
compartment syndrome
compatible
compensation
  cardiac
  cardiac gating
  respiratory
compensatory emphysema
competent ileocecal valve
complete dislocation
complex
  Eisenmenger
  Ghon
  primary
complicated dislocation
component
compound dislocation
compound fracture
compound presentation
compression fracture

compression of breast
compression plate and screws
Compton effect
Compuscan Hittman computerized electrocardioscanner
computed axial tomography (CAT) scan
computed sonography, Acuson
computed tomography dose index (CTDI)
computed transmission tomography
computerized (or computed) tomography (CT)
computerized transverse axial tomography (CTAT)
concatenation
concave, concavity
concentric contraction
concentric hourglass stenosis
concentric plaque
concha, inferior nasal
conduit, ileal
condylarthrosis
condylar fracture
condylar split fracture
condyle
   external
   lateral
   medial
condyloid joint
coned-down appearance of colon
coned-down view
coned view
configuration, mitral
confluence of sinuses
confluent infiltrate
congenital anomaly
congenital biliary atresia
congenital deformity
congenital dilatation of intrahepatic bile duct
congenital dislocation

congenital dysplasia of hip (CDH)
congenital intercalary limb absence
congenital laryngeal atresia
congenital malrotation of the gut
congenital megacolon
congenital terminal limb absence
congestion, pulmonary vascular
congestive heart failure (CHF)
conglomerate calcification
conjugata vera
conjugate diameter
conjugate, true
connective tubing
Conray contrast medium
consecutive dislocation
consolidation
   homogeneous acinar
   nonhomogeneous
   patchy
consolidative process
constant, Planck
constriction, hourglass
contiguous
continuity of bone
continuous wave
contour, diaphragmatic
contraction
   cicatricial
   concentric
   peristaltic
   tertiary
contralateral
contrast
   bolus of
   clearance of
   collection of
   column of
   enhanced
   enhancement of
   extravasated
   excretion of
   ferromagnetic

contrast *(cont.)*
  film
  high
  intravenous (I.V.)
  injection of
  iodinated
  leakage of
  long-scale
  low
  lymphangiographic
  nonionic
  oral
  paradoxical hyperconcentration
    of
  poor visualization of
  prompt excretion of
  prompt visualization of
  reaction to
  refluxed
  residual
  resolution of
  retention of
  sonicated
  visualization of
contrast agent
contrast bolus
contrast column
contrast enhancement
contrast extravasation
contrast-filled stomach
contrast injection
contrast medium (pl. media)
  (also see *radioisotope*)
  Amipaque
  Angio-Conray
  Angiografin
  Angiovist 282; 292; 370
  Baricon
  barium sulfate
  Baro-CAT
  Baroflave
  Barosperse 110

contrast medium *(cont.)*
  Biligrafin
  Biliscopin
  Bilivist
  Bilopaque
  bunamiodyl (also buniodyl)
  Cardiografin sodium
  Cholebrine
  Cholografin meglumine
  Conray-30; -43; -60; -325; -400
  Cr-HIDA
  Cysto-Conray II
  Cystografin
  Cystokon
  diatrizoate meglumine
  diatrizoate sodium
  Diodrast
  Dionosil
  diprotrizoate
  Duografin
  Ethiodol
  Gastrografin
  Gastrovist
  Gd-DTPA
  Hexabrix
  Hippuran
  Hipputope
  Hypaque-76
  Hypaque-Cysto
  Hypaque-M
  Hypaque meglumine
  Hypaque sodium
  Intropaque
  iobenzamic acid
  iocarmic acid
  iocetamic acid
  iodamide
  iodamine meglumine
  iodipamide meglumine
  iodohippurate sodium
  iodomethamate sodium
  iodophthalein sodium

contrast medium *(cont.)*
- iodopyracet
- Iodotope
- iohexol
- iopamidol
- iopanoic acid
- iopentol
- iophendylate
- iopydol
- iopydone
- iosefamic acid
- iotetric acid
- iothalamate meglumine; sodium
- iotrol
- iotroxic acid
- ioversol
- ioxaglate meglumine
- ioxaglate sodium
- ipodate calcium
- ipodate sodium
- Isopaque
- Isovue-300; -370
- Isovue-M 200; 300
- Kinevac
- Lipiodol
- Liquipake
- Lymphazurin
- Magnevist
- MD-50; MD-60; MD-76
- MD-Gastroview
- MDP
- methiodal sodium
- metrizamide
- MIBG (metaiodobenzyl-guanidine)
- Niopam
- Novopaque
- Omnipaque
- Optiray
- Orabilix sodium
- Oragrafin calcium
- Oragrafin sodium
- Pantopaque

contrast medium *(cont.)*
- Perchloracap
- pertechnetate sodium
- Phentetiothalein
- Priodax
- propyliodone
- Renografin-60; -76
- Reno-M-Dip; M-30; M-60
- Renovist II
- Renovue-Dip; -65
- Salpix
- SHU-454
- Sinografin
- Skiodan
- sodium iodide
- sodium iodomethamate
- sodium pertechnetate
- Solu-Biloptin
- SPP (superparamagnetic particle)
- Telepaque
- Thixokon
- Thorotrast
- Tomocat
- tyropanoate sodium
- Tyropaque
- Ultravist
- Urografin
- Urovist Cysto
- Urovist meglumine; sodium
- Vascoray
- ZK44012

contrast resolution

contrast-to-noise (C/N) ratio

contrast ventriculography

contrecoup fracture

contusion
- pulmonary
- soft tissue

conus arteriosus

conus medullaris

converter
- analog to digital (A to D)

converter *(cont.)*
    digital to analog (D to A)
convex linear array
convexity
convolution, Arnold
convolution of Gratiolet
coordinates (X, Y, and Z) for target
    lesion
COPD (chronic obstructive
    pulmonary disease)
Cope nephrostomy tube
Cope point
co-precipitation
coprolith
coprostasis
cor pulmonale
cor triatriatum
coracoclavicular ligament complex
coracoid notch
coracoid process of scapula
coracoid tuberosity
cord
    spinal
    vocal
cordate pelvis
cordis atrium
corkscrew esophagus
cornu, cornua
coronal image, multi-echo
coronal orientation
coronal plane
coronal projection
coronal section
coronal suture
coronal view
corona radiata
coronary angiogram
    left (LCA)
    right (RCA)
coronary artery
coronary artery bypass graft
    (CABG)

coronary cineangiography
coronary occlusion
coronary sulcus
coronoid fossa
coronoid process of mandible
coronoid process of ulna
corpora fornicis
corpora restiformia
corpus callosum
corpus sterni
corpus striatum
corpus uteri
correlation
    clinical
    histologic
correlation time
cortex, articular
cortical hyperostosis, infantile
cortical necrosis
cortical signet ring shadow
cortical sulci
cortical thumb
cortices (pl. of cortex)
corticocallosal dysgenesis
corticomedullary
costa fluctuans decima
costae spuriae
costae verae
costal angle
costal bone
costal cartilage
costal margin
costal notch
costal process
costal sulcus
costal tubercle
costochondral junction
costoclavicular
costophrenic (CP) angle, blunted
costophrenic septal lines
costosternal angle
costovertebral angle

Cotrel-Dubousset spinal instru-
mentation
cottage loaf appearance
Cotton ankle fracture
cotyloid notch
coulomb (C)
Coumadin
Councill catheter
counter-current aortography
counter, proportional
course of ureter
course of vessel
coursing of gas
Courvoisier gallbladder
coxa adducta
coxa flexa
coxa plana
coxa valga
coxa vara deformity of hip
coxa vara luxans
coxarthritis
coxarthropathy
coxitis, senile
CP (costophrenic) angle
CPA (cerebellopontile or cerebellopontine angle)
CPD (cephalopelvic disproportion)
cranial angulation, AP projection
cranial suture
cranial trauma
cranial view
craniocaudad projection
craniocaudal view
craniofacial disjunction
craniofacial dysostosis
craniolacunia
craniopathy
craniosclerosis
craniotomy
cranium, cranial
crater, ulcer
crescent of the cardia

crescent-shaped fibrocartilaginous
disk
crest, iliac
Cr-HIDA contrast medium
cribriform bone
cribriform plate
cribriform process
cricoarytenoid
cricoid cartilage
cricopharyngeal diverticulum
crisscross heart
crista galli
crista iliaca
crista pubica
crista sacralis lateralis
crista vestibuli
Crohn disease
crossed-coil design
cross-filling
cross-sectional zone
cross-table lateral film
Crouzon disease
crowding of bronchovascular
markings
cruciate incision
cruciate ligament
cruciatum cruris ligament
crura cerebri
crushed bone
crushing-type injury
crus of the diaphragm
cryomagnet
cryostat
crypt, Luschka
crypt of Lieberkühn
crypt of Morgagni
CSF (cerebrospinal fluid)
CT (cardiothoracic) ratio
CT (computerized tomography)
CT cisternogram, metrizamide
(MCTC)
CT gantry

CT scan, dual energy
CT scan with contrast enhancement
CT sialography
CT stereotaxic guide, BRW
CT scanner
   cine
   GE CT/T 8800
   Somatom DR
CTAT (computerized transverse
   axial tomography)
CTDI (computed tomography dose
   index)
cubic centimeter (cc)
cubital fossa
cubital tunnel syndrome
cubitus valgus deformity
cubitus varus deformity
cuboid bone
cuffing, peribronchial
cul-de-sac of Douglas
cuneiform bone of carpus
cup
   hip replacement
   prosthesis
cup-and-spill stomach
cupula, diaphragmatic
curie (Ci)
current, pulsing
curvature
   cervical
   dorsal kyphotic
   flattening of normal lordotic
   greater
   humpbacked spinal
   lesser
   lumbar
   normal cervical
   radius of
curve
   Bragg
   sigmoid
   time-density

curvilinear calcification
Cushing ulcer
cutaneopancreatic
cut-biopsy needle (see *needle)*
cutdown
cutoff
cuts, tomographic
CVA (cerebrovascular accident)
CVA (costovertebral angle)
CVP (central venous pressure) line
cyanocobalamin radioactive agent
cylindroma
cyllosis
cyst
   dermoid
   endodermal
   hemorrhagic
   ovarian
   renal
cyst in acetabulum
cystic astrocytoma
cystic change
cystic duct cholangiogram
cystic fibrosis
cystic lesion, sonolucent
cystic mazoplasia
cystic neoplasm
cystic osteofibromatosis
cystocele, protrusion of
Cysto-Conray II contrast medium
Cystografin contrast medium
cystogram, -graphy
   delayed
   excretory
   postvoiding
   radionuclide
   retrograde
   triple voiding
   voiding
cystoscopic urography
cystourethrogram, voiding (VCUG)
Cytomel suppression

# D, d

dactyl
Dagradi classification of esophageal
 varices
DALM (dysplasia with associated
 lesion or mass)
dance, hilar
Dance sign
Dandy-Walker syndrome
date, menstrual
DBM (demineralized bone matrix)
DCBE (double contrast barium
 enema)
dead time
debris
 bone
 particulate
De Broglie wavelength
decay
 beta
 exponential
decay series
decompensation, cardiac
decortication
decrease in echo signal on
 ultrasound
decreased uptake of iodine
decubitus position
decubitus view
deep-shelled acetabulum
deep venous channel
deep venous thrombosis
defecation
defecogram, -graphy
defect
 aorticopulmonary septal
 atrial septal
 atrioseptal
 bridging of

defect *(cont.)*
 cauliflower-shaped
 chain of lakes filling
 cold
 cortical
 developmental
 discoid filling
 extradural
 filling
 frondlike filling
 fusiform
 hot
 lucent
 mapping of
 nonsubperiosteal cortical
 osseous
 ostium primum
 osteochondral
 polypoid filling
 segmental
 soft tissue
 subcortical
 subperiosteal cortical
 trochlear
 ventral hernia
 ventricular septal
deficiency disease
deficit, perfusion
deformity
 Akerlund
 angular
 back-knee
 biconcave
 bifid thumb
 bony
 boutonniere (of finger)
 bowing
 bunion

deformity *(cont.)*
  buttonhole
  cavovarus
  chain of lakes
  clawfoot
  clawhand
  clawtoe
  cloverleaf
  codfish
  compensatory
  congenital vertical talus foot
  coxa vara
  cubitus valgus
  cubitus varus
  duodenal bulb
  equinovalgus
  eversion-external rotation
  flexion
  funnel
  genu valgum
  genu varum
  gun stock
  hallux flexus
  hallux malleus
  hallux rigidus
  hallux valgus
  hallux varus
  hatchet-head
  Hill-Sachs
  hourglass
  Ilfeld-Holder
  internal rotation
  intrinsic minus
  intrinsic plus
  joint
  mallet finger
  metatarsus adductocavus
  metatarsus adductovarus
  metatarsus adductus
  metatarsus atavicus
  metatarsus latus
  metatarsus primus varus

deformity *(cont.)*
  metatarsus varus
  pectus excavatum
  phrygian cap
  pigeon breast
  plantar flexion-inversion
  recurvatum
  rotational
  silver-fork
  Sprengel
  swan-neck finger
  trefoil
  triphalangeal thumb
  trigger finger
  ulnar drift
  valgus
  varus
  Volkmann
  wedging
  Whitehead
degenerative arthritic change
degenerative change
degenerative disease
degenerative spur, spurring
deglutition
deglutition mechanism
delayed CT scan
delay in excretory phase, marked
demilune
demineralization of bone
demineralized bone matrix (DBM)
demodulator
dendritic lesion
dens (odontoid process of axis)
dens view of cervical spine
densitometry test
  dual photon
  single photon
density
  abdominal soft tissue
  bands of
  calcific

density *(cont.)*
    calcified
    homogeneous
    ill-defined
    increased bone
    linear
    linear increased
    metallic
    mottled
    nodular
    parenchymal
    patchy
    pleural
    pulmonary
    radiographic
    radiolucent
    radiopaque
    retroareolar
    ropy
    soft tissue
    spin
dentate line
dentate nucleus
dentate suture
Denver hydrocephalus shunt
Denver peritoneal venous shunt
deossification
dephasing
deposition, calcium
depressed fracture
depression of fragment
de Quervain disease
derangement
derby hat fracture
dermoid cyst
dermoid tumor
derotation
DES (diffuse esophageal spasm)
Desault fracture
descending aorta
descending colon
descending duodenum

descensus
Desilets-Hoffman introducer
detector array
detector, Doppler blood flow
Deutschländer's disease
Deventer diameter
device
    fixation
    intramedullary fixation
    metallic long screw fixation
    plate-and-screw fixation
dextrocardia
dextrogastria
dextroposition of aorta
dextrorotatory
dextrorotoscoliosis
dextroscoliosis
dextrotropic
diacondylar fracture
diagnosis, differential
diagnostic
diagonal conjugate diameter
diamagnetic shift
diametaphyseal
diametaphysis
diameter
    AP
    Baudelocque
    bi-ischial
    biparietal (BPD)
    coccygeopubic
    conjugate
    Deventer
    diagonal conjugate
    intercristal
    internal conjugate
    intertuberal
    Lohlein
    pelvic
    sacropubic
    transverse
    transverse pelvic

diaphragm
  crus of
  leaf of
  tenting of
diaphragmatically directed
  chest tube
diaphragmatic contour
diaphragmatic cupula
diaphragmatic hernia
diaphyseal dysplasia
diaphyseal fracture
diaphyseal sclerosis
diaphysis
diastasis, sutural
diastatic fracture
diatrizoate meglumine contrast
  medium
diatrizoate sodium contrast medium
didactylism
didelphia
differential diagnosis
differentiated
diffuse, diffusion
diffuse enlargement of thyroid
diffuse idiopathic sclerosis hyperostosis (DISH)
diffuse progressive ossifying polymyositis
diffuse stippled calcification
digestion
digestive tract
digestive system
digit
digital frequency analysis
digital imaging
digital subtraction angiography
  (DSA)
digital vascular imaging (DVI)
digital videoangiography
Digitron DVI/DSA computer
digitus pedis

dilatation
  anal
  aneurysmal
  bowel
  cardiac
  ductal
  esophageal
  fusiform
  gastric
  periportal sinusoidal
  pneumatic bag esophageal
  prognathous
dilate
dilated extrahepatic bile ducts
dilated intrahepatic biliary radicles
dilated loops of bowel
dilation, dilatation
  biliary
  esophageal
  extrahepatic biliary cystic
  hepatic web
  percutaneous balloon
  pneumatic balloon catheter
dilator
  Amplatz
  Vance
dimension, axial
dimetria
diminution
Diodrast contrast medium
Dionosil contrast medium
DIP (distal interphalangeal) joint
dipolar interaction
diprotrizoate contrast medium
dipyridamole echocardiography test
dipyridamole handgrip test
dipyridamole infusion test
dipyridamole thallium 201 scintigraphy
dipyridamole thallium scan
dipyridamole thallium ventriculography

direct fracture
direct hernia
direction, aboral
disc (see *disk*)
discoid filling defect
discoid lateral meniscus
discrepancy, leg length
discrete mass
discriminator
disease
  active
  Addison
  air-space
  Albers-Schönberg
  Albert
  Alzheimer
  amyloid
  Aran-Duchenne
  atherosclerotic
  Bamberger-Marie
  Banti
  Beau
  Beauvais
  Bekhterev
  bilateral iliac
  Blount
  Bonfil
  Bouchard
  Brinton
  Brodie
  Bruck
  Budlinger-Ludlof-Laewen
  Busquet
  Caffey
  Calvé-Perthes
  Camurati-Engelmann
  cardiopulmonary
  Caroli
  Charcot-Marie-Tooth
  Chester
  chronic
  chronic lung

disease *(cont.)*
  COPD (chronic obstructive
    pulmonary disease)
  Crohn
  Crouzon
  deficiency
  degenerative
  de Quervain
  Deutschländer
  Duroziez
  emphysematous
  Engel-Recklinghausen
  Erb
  Fahr-Volhard
  Favre
  Fenwick
  Fleischner
  Forestier
  Freiberg
  Gamna
  Gandy-Nanta
  Gee-Herter
  Glénard
  granulomatous
  Gull
  Hagner
  Hand-Schüller-Christian
  Hashimoto
  Heberden
  Henderson-Jones
  hepatic venous web
  Hirschsprung
  Hodgkin
  Hoffa
  Huppert
  hyaline membrane
  inflammatory
  Jaffe-Lichtenstein
  Jansen
  juvenile Paget
  Kahler
  Kashin-Beck

disease *(cont.)*
- Kienböck
- Köhler
- Köhler-Pellegrini-Stieda
- Kugelberg-Welander
- Kümmell
- Lane
- Larsen
- Larsen-Johansson
- Legg
- Legg-Calvé
- Legg-Calvé-Perthes
- Legg-Calvé-Waldenström
- Legg-Perthes
- MacLean-Maxwell
- Marie
- Marie-Bamberger
- Marie-Strümpell
- Marie-Tooth
- Martin
- Meige
- metastatic
- Miller
- Milroy
- Münchmeyer
- Niemann-Pick
- obstructive lung
- Ollier
- Osgood-Schlatter
- Paas
- Paget
- patchy
- Payr
- Pel-Ebstein
- Pellegrini
- Pellegrini-Stieda
- peptic ulcer (PUD)
- peripheral lung
- Petit
- Pick
- Preiser
- pulmonary

disease *(cont.)*
- Quervain (de Quervain)
- Recklinghausen (of bone)
- renal parenchymal
- reversible obstructive airways
- rheumatic valvular
- Ruysch
- sacroiliac
- Schanz
- Scheuermann
- Schlatter-Osgood
- Schmorl
- Schüller
- Sever
- Sternberg
- Still
- Strümpell
- Strümpell-Marie
- Sturge-Weber
- Sudeck
- Swediaur
- Thiemann
- underlying
- Vaquez
- Volkmann
- von Gierke
- von Recklinghausen
- Waldenström
- Wegner
- widespread

dishpan fracture
DISI (dorsal intercalary segment instability)
DISIDA scan
disintegration
disk (or disc)
- bulging
- crescent-shaped fibrocartilaginous
- herniated
- intervertebral
- lumbar
- lumbosacral

disk bulge; bulging
disk fragment
disk herniation
disk interspace
disk margin
disk protrusion
disk space narrowing
diskectomy, percutaneous automated
diskectomy with Cloward fusion
dislocation
   anterior hip
   anterior-inferior
   anterior temporomandibular
   ankle
   Bell-Dally cervical
   boutonnière hand
   bursting
   carpal lunate
   carpometacarpal
   central
   Chopart ankle
   closed
   complete
   complicated
   compound
   congenital (of the hip) (CDH)
   consecutive
   divergent elbow
   fracture
   frank
   gamekeeper's
   glenohumeral joint
   habitual
   incomplete
   intrathoracic (of shoulder)
   intrauterine
   irreducible
   isolated
   Kienböck
   knee
   Lisfranc
   lunate

dislocation *(cont.)*
   luxatio erecta shoulder
   metacarpophalangeal
   milkmaid's elbow
   Monteggia
   Nélaton ankle
   nonreducible
   old
   open
   Otto pelvis
   partial
   pathologic
   perilunate carpal
   posterior hip
   primitive
   radial head
   recent
   recurrent
   scapholunate
   simple
   Smith
   subastragalar
   subcoracoid (of shoulder)
   subglenoid (of shoulder)
   subspinous
   talar
   tarsal
   tarsometatarsal
   tibiotarsal
   transradial styloid perilunate
   transscaphoid perilunate
   traumatic
   triquetrolunate
   vertebral
   volar semilunar wrist
dislocation fracture
dislocation of atlas, nontraumatic
displacement
disproportion, cephalopelvic (CPD)
disruption
   bony
   joint
   ligamentous

disruption of pancreatic duct
dissecans
   osteochondritis
   osteochondrosis
dissect, dissection
dissecting aneurysm
dissection, aortic
disseminated
distal fundal portion of the
   gallbladder
distal interphalangeal (DIP) joint
distally
distal phalanx
distal portion of the gastric antrum
distal splenorenal shunt (DSRS)
distal third of the thoracic
   esophagus
distend, distention
distention
   abdominal
   colonic
   gaseous
   gastric
   intestinal
   postprandial
   rectal
distraction of fracture
distribution
   Boltzmann
   gaussian
   inhomogeneous tracer
   mottled
   uniform
disturbance, functional
disuse osteoporosis
divergent dislocation
diverticulitis
diverticulosis
diverticulum, diverticula
   colonic
   cricopharyngeal
   epiphrenic

diverticulum *(cont.)*
   esophageal
   false
   functional
   Ganser
   Graser
   hepatic
   hypopharyngeal
   IDD (intraluminal duodenal)
   intestinal
   intraluminal duodenal (IDD)
   intramural
   juxtapapillary
   Kirchner
   Meckel
   midesophageal
   perforated
   periampullary
   pharyngoesophageal
   Rokitansky
   traction
   Vater
   vesical
   Zenker
diverticulum of Nuck
Dobbhoff tube
dolichocephaly
dolichocolon
dolichoesophagus
dolichosigmoid
dome of the bladder
dome of the liver
dome of the urinary bladder
Doppler blood flow velocity signal
Doppler flow signal
Doppler frequency shift
Doppler, real-time Color Flow
Doppler ultrasound
dorsal capsule
dorsal position
dorsal recumbent position
dorsal spine

dorsiflexion
dorsoanterior
dorsocephalad
dorsolateral
dorsoposterior
dorsum, dorsal
dorsum pedis
dose
    absorbed
    median lethal
    multiple scan average (MSAD)
dose index, computed tomography
    (CTDI)
dosimeter
dosimetry, therminoluminescent
Dos Santos needle
Dotter-Judkins technique
double-bubble duodenal sign
double contrast barium enema
    (DCBE)
double contrast roentgenography
double contrast study
double contrast visualization
double fracture
double photon absorptiometry
    (DPA)
double tracking of barium
Douglas, cul-de-sac of
dowager's hump
DPA (double photon absorp-
    tiometry)
drain
    Castaneda internal-external
    Penrose
    subphrenic
drainage tube
draining sinus
drop finger
dropfoot
dropsy
DSA (digital subtraction angi-
    ography), intra-arterial

DSRS (distal splenorenal shunt)
DTPA renography
dual contrast study
dual photon densitometry test for
    osteoporosis
duct
    accessory pancreatic
    beaded hepatic
    bile
    biliary
    Botallo
    common
    common bile (CBD)
    common hepatic
    cystic
    distal bile
    extrahepatic bile
    fusiform widening of
    gall
    Gartner
    hepatic
    Hering
    interlobular bile
    intrahepatic biliary
    main pancreatic (MPD)
    middle extrahepatic bile
    normal caliber
    pancreatic
    perilobular
    preampullary portion of bile
    prepapillary bile
    Santorini
    Stensen
    subvesical
    terminal bile
    Vater
    vitelline
    Wirsung
    wolffian
duct of Santorini
duct of Vater
duct of Wirsung

ductal ectasia
ductal hyperplasia
ductal pattern
ductular
ductule
ductus arteriosus
dumbbell-shaped shadow
dumping stomach syndrome
duodenal atresia
duodenal bulb
duodenal cap
duodenal C-loop
duodenal duplication
duodenal impression on liver
duodenal loop
duodenal papilla
duodenal sweep
duodenal terminus
duodenal tumor, periampullary
duodenal ulcer
duodenitis
   chronic atrophic
   erosive
duodenogastric reflux
duodenogastroscopy, retrograde
  (RDG)
duodenography, hypotonic
duodenopancreatic reflux
duodenum
   descending
   distal
   first portion of
   second portion of
   supravaterian
   third portion of
duodenum deformed by scarring
Duografin contrast medium
duplex Doppler scan

duplex Doppler sonography (DS)
duplex pulsed-Doppler sonography
duplication, duodenal
Dupuytren fracture
Duverney fracture
dural impingement
dural puncture
dural sac
Duroziez disease
DVI (digital vascular imaging)
dynamic computerized tomography
  (CT)
dynode
dysarthrosis
dyschezia
dyschondroplasia
dyscrasic fracture
dyskinesia, biliary
dysmotility, esophageal
dysostosis
   cleidocranial
   craniofacial
   metaphyseal
dyspepsia, dyspeptic
dysphagia
dysplasia
   arteriohepatic
   fibrous
   polypoid
   retroareolar
   sheetlike
dysplasia with associated lesion
  or mass (DALM)
dysplastic
dyspnea
dystocia
dystopia, dystopic

# E, e

E sign
EBA (extrahepatic biliary atresia)
eburnation
eccentric plaque
eccentric pyloric channel
ECG-synchronized digital subtraction angiography
echo, echoes
 internal
 solid
echocardiography
 color flow imaging Doppler
 contrast
 contrast-enhanced
 cross-sectional
 CW (continuous wave) Doppler
 intracoronary contrast
 myocardial contrast (MCE)
 myocardial perfusion
 postcontrast
 precontrast
 sector scan
 two-dimensional (2-D)
echo characteristics
echodense
echogenic renal parenchyma
echogenic solid lesion or mass
echogenicity
echography, renal
echoic
echo pattern
 homogeneous
 inhomogeneous
echo planar imaging
echo texture
echo time (TE)
ECMO (extracorporeal membrane
 oxygenation) therapy

ectasia, ductal
ectatic
ectocardia
ectopic pregnancy
ectrodactyly
eddies (pl. of eddy)
eddy current
edema
 alveolar
 antral
 bullous-like
 collateral
 diffuse
 focal
 interstitial
 nerve root
 patchy
 pericholecystic
 liver
 pulmonary
edematous
edge, sawtooth
efface, effacement
effect
 Compton
 halo
 mass
efferent view
effluent
effort, inspiratory
effusion
 cardiac
 free pleural
 joint
 loculated
 pericardial
 pleural
EG (esophagogastric) junction

Egan technique
eggshell border of aneurysm
eggshell-like
Eisenmenger complex
ejecta
ejection fraction, left ventricular
Ektascan laser printer
elbow
    pulled
    tennis
electrocardiogram, -graph
electrode
    mini EKG
    monitoring
electrogastrogram, -graphy
electrometer
electrophoresis
element, posterior
elevation
ellipsoid joint
elongation of aorta
elongation of colon
Elscint CT scanner
elutriation
embolic phenomenon
embolism, pulmonary
embolization
    angiographic variceal
    transcatheter variceal
    transhepatic (THE)
embolus, pulmonary
embryonal cell carcinoma
embryonic
emesis
EMI CT scanner
eminence
    arcuate
    collateral
    hypothenar
    iliopectineal
    intercondyloid
    thenar

emphysema
    bullous
    compensatory
    obstructive
    subcutaneous
    substantial
emphysematous disease
emphysematous gastritis
emptying time
empty sella syndrome
empyema of gallbladder
enarthrosis
encapsulated
encase
encephalomalacia
enchondral ossification
enchondroma
enchondromatosis
encroach
encroachment, bony
endobronchial
endocardial fibroelastosis
endocarditis
endocardium
endochondral bone
endochondral ossification
endocrine fracture
endodermal cyst
endoergic reaction
endogenous callus formation
endometrial echo
endometriosis, studding of
endopericarditis
endoscopic retrograde cholangio-
    pancreatography (ERCP)
endoscopic retrograde pancreatic
    duct cannulation
endoscopic ultrasonography (EUS)
endosteal callus
endosteal surface
endotracheal (ET) tube
endplate of vertebral body

enema
  air contrast barium
  barium
  double contrast barium (DCBE)
  full column barium
energy decays
energy, kinetic
en face ("in front") view
Engel-Recklinghausen disease
enhanced CAT scan
enhancement
  contrast
  nonhomogeneous
enlargement, cardiac
ensiform appendix
ensiform process
enteritis, cicatrizing
enterocystoma
enterolith
enteron
enteroptosis
entrap
entry zone
epactal
epicondyle, epicondylar
epicondylitis
  lateral
  medial
epicranial aponeurosis
epidural blood
epidural space
epigastric hernia
epigastrium
epiglottis
epiphrenic
epiphrenic diverticulum
epiphyseal arrest
epiphyseal chondroblastic growth
epiphyseal coxa vara
epiphyseal fracture
epiphyseal hyperplasia
epiphyseal plate

epiphysiodesis
epiphysis (pl. epiphyses)
  capital femoral
  capitular
  stippled
  tibial
epiphysitis of calcaneus
epiploic
epiploitis
epiploon (the omentum)
epithalamus
epitrochlea, epitrochlear
equation
  Bloch
  Larmor
  Stewart-Hamilton
equilibrium radionuclide angiogram
equipment, real-time
Erb disease
ERCP (endoscopic retrograde
  cholangiopancreatography)
erect position
erect view
erosion
  duodenal
  gastric antral
  linear
  salt and pepper duodenal
erosive gastritis
esophageal A ring
esophageal atresia
esophageal B ring
esophageal clearing
esophageal dilatation
esophageal diverticulum
esophageal dysmotility
esophageal fold
esophageal hiatus
esophageal inlet
esophageal motility
esophageal reflux
esophageal spasm, intermittent

esophageal stricture
esophageal web
esophagitis, reflux (RE)
esophagogastric (EG) junction
esophagogram
esophagojejunostomy
esophagram
esophagus
  Barrett
  cervical
  columnar-lined
  corkscrew
  distal
  dysmotile
  nutcracker
  spastic
  thoracic
  tortuous
  upper thoracic
Essex-Lopresti calcaneal fracture
ESWL (extracorporeal shock wave lithotripsy)
ET (endotracheal) tube
Ethiodane contrast medium
ethiodized oil
Ethiodol contrast medium
ethmoid bone
ethmoid sinus
etiology
EUS (endoscopic ultrasonography)
euthyroid
evacuation disorder
evacuation, precipitate
Evans classification of inter-trochanteric fracture
eventration of diaphragm
eversion
Ewald test meal
Ewing tumor
exchange
  coupling
  ion
excrescence, bony

excrete, excretion
excretory urogram
exercise, modified stage
exhalation
Exner plexus
exocardia
exoccipital bone
exoergic reaction
exogenous callus formation
exogenous obesity
exostosis, bony
expanded lung
expiration
expiratory chest
exponential decay
exstrophy
extension
  Buck
  Codivilla
extension injury of spine
external condyle
external iliac artery
external jugular system
extirpation
extra-articular fracture
extracapsular fracture
extracorporeal membrane oxygenation (ECMO) therapy
extradural defect
extrahepatic bile ducts, dilated
extrahepatic biliary atresia (EBA)
extraperitoneal rupture
extrapleural
extrathecal
extrauterine gestation
extrauterine pregnancy
extravasation of contrast
extravasation of dye
extravasation of joint fluid
extrinsic compression
extubation, interval
exudate, exudative
E-Z-Paque barium suspension

# F, f

fabella
facet, articular
facet dislocation of cervical spine
facet joint, posterior
facies ossea
factor
   Boltzmann
   geometry
   technical
Fahr-Volhard disease
failure
   cardiac
   ventricular
falcine region
falcula, falcular
fallopian tube
Fallot, tetralogy of
false color scale
false diverticulum
false-negative result
false-positive result
falx cerebelli
falx cerebri
familial avascular necrosis of
   phalangeal epiphysis
familial osteoarthropathy of fingers
fan beam
Faraday shield
fascia, lateroconal
fascial tract
fasciculus cerebrospinalis
fasciculus cuneatus
fasciculus dorsolateralis
fasciculus occipitofrontalis
fast Fourier spectral analysis
fast Fourier transform (FFT)
fat
   abdominal

fat *(cont.)*
   preperitoneal
   properitoneal
   protruding
   subcutaneous
fatigue fracture
fat line, subcutaneous
fat pad
   abdominal
   pericardial
fat plane
fatty meal sonogram (FMS)
faveolate
Favre disease
FB (foreign body)
fecalith
fecal material, retained
fecaloid
fecaloma
fecal residue
feces, inspissation of
Fe-Ex orogastric tube magnet
felon
femoral aortic flush catheter
femoral artery
femoral bone
femoral condyle
femoral head
femoral hernia
femoral neck
femoral tuberosity
femoral vein
femoral visceral renal curve catheter
femorotibial
femtoliter (fL)
femur length
femur, femoral
fenestration, aorticopulmonary

Fenwick disease
ferromagnetic relaxation
fetal lobulation
fetal motion; movement
fetal placenta
fetal small parts
fetometry
fetuses (pl. of fetus)
fetus, intrauterine
FFT (fast Fourier transform)
fiberoptic bronchoscopy (FOB)
fiberscope, Olympus GF-EU1 ultra-
    sound
fibrocalcific, fibrocalcification
fibrocartilage
fibrocartilaginous disk
fibrocartilaginous plate
fibrocystic residual
fibroid
    calcified
    uterine
fibroid uterus
fibrolipoma
fibroma
    aponeurotic
    chondromyxoid
    nonossifying
    ossifying
    osteogenic
    periosteal
fibromuscular dysplasia
fibromyoma
fibronodular
fibrosarcoma
fibrosis
    basilar
    diffuse interstitial
    interstitial
    perihilar
    pulmonary
fibro-osseous tunnel

fibrosis
    cystic
    diffuse interstitial
    interstitial
    postradiation
fibrotic residual
fibrotic tissue
fibrous dysplasia
fibrous dysplasia ossificans
    progressiva
fibrous nonunion
fibrous syndesmosis
fibrous union
fibula, fibular
fibular bone
fibular notch
Fick equation
FID (free induction decay)
field
    lower lung
    lung
    midlung
    upper lung
field gradient
field lock
field of view (FOV)
filiform appendix
fill and spill of dye (in fallopian
    tubes)
filling defect (see *defect)*
filling factor
filling of a vessel
film, x-ray (see also *view)*
    AP (anteroposterior)
    chiropractic
    comparison
    cross-table lateral
    expiratory
    flat plate
    high-contrast
    lateral
    lateral decubitus

film *(cont.)*
  limited
  low-contrast
  low-dose
  oblique
  outside
  overhead
  PA (posteroanterior)
  plain
  portable
  postevacuation
  postvoid(ing)
  preliminary
  prone
  scout
  sequential
  serial
  skull
  spot
  stress
  subtraction
  upright
  working
filtered-back projection
filter, wall
filum terminale
fimbriated end of fallopian tube
fine calcification
fine needle
fine-needle biopsy
finger
  drop
  index
  little
  long
  mallet
  ring
fingertip lesion
first-pass effect
first-pass view
fish-scale gallbladder
fission

fissura cerebri lateralis
fissura congenita
fissure
  auricular
  calcarine
  longitudinal
  occipital
  palpebral
fissure fracture
fissure of Rolando
fissure of Sylvius
fistula
  colovesical
  gastric
  Mann-Bollman
  retroperitoneal
  tracheo-esophageal
  vesicovaginal
fistulogram, -graphy
fistulous formation
fistulous tract
fixation device, plate-and-screw
fixation, open reduction and
  internal (ORIF)
fixed segment of bowel
fL (femtoliter)
flaccid     FLAIR - fluid attenue
flail chest          imaging
flank bone (ilium)
flare of the condyles
FLASH (fast low-angle shot)
  cardiac MRI
flat bone
flatfoot
flat pelvis
flat plate of abdomen
flattening of fornix
flatulence
flatus
flavum, ligamentum
Flechsig tract
Fleischer disease

Fleischmann bursa
flexion and extension
flexion deformity
flexion-distraction injury of spine
flexion injury of spine
flexion maneuver
flexion-rotation injury of spine
FlexStrand cable
flexure
   hepatic
   splenic
flip angle
flocculation on barium enema
floor, bladder
flow
   antegrade bile
   antegrade blood
   cerebral brain
   physiologic
   retrograde
flow scan
flow study
fluctuant mass
fluid
   amniotic
   cerebrospinal
   free abdominal
   interstitial
   pelvic
   pericardial
   pleural
   synovial
fluid level
fluid wave
fluorescein angiography
fluorescence
fluoroscope, mobile
fluoroscopic assistance
fluoroscopic control, advanced
   under
fluoroscopic guidance
fluoroscopic view

fluoroscopy, C-arm
flush aortogram, -graphy
FMS (fatty meal sonogram)
focal abnormality
focal edema
focal stenosis
focus, foci
fog or fogging effect on CT
Fogarty balloon biliary catheter
Fogarty Hydrogrip clamp
fold
   cecal
   cholecystoduodenocolic
   Douglas
   duodenojejunal
   duodenomesocolic
   epigastric
   esophageal
   flattened duodenal
   gastric
   gastropancreatic
   gluteal
   haustral
   Hensing
   hepatopancreatic
   ileocolic
   Kerckring
   Kohlrausch
   Nélaton
   palatopharyngeal
   prepyloric
   rectal
   rugal
   semilunar
   sentinel
   sigmoid
   thickened
folded fundus gallbladder
follicle, follicles
   aggregated
   graafian
   intestinal

follow-through, small-bowel
follow-up (n., adj.), follow up (v.)
fontanelle
foot
   Charcot
   Friedreich
   reel
footling presentation
foramen
   Botallo
   great sacrosciatic
   sacrosciatic
foramen caecum
foramen magnum
foramen obturatum
foramen of Bochdalek
foramen of Luschka
foramen of Magendie
foramen of Monro
foramen of Morgagni
foramen of Winslow
foramen ovale
foramen ovale lacerum
foramen rotundum
foramen spinosum
foramina (pl. of foramen)
foramina, intervertebral
foraminal space
forearm
forefoot, mid- and
foreign body (FB)
   metallic
   tracheobronchial
Forestier disease
formation
   bat-wing
   callus
   fistulous
   Gothic arch
   marginal osteophyte
   osteophyte
   saccular
   spur

fornices (pl. of fornix)
fornix cerebri
fornix, flattening of
forward subluxation
fossa
   anconeal (also anconal)
   antecubital
   coronoid
   cubital
   Gruber
   hyaloid
   iliac
   intercondyloid
   infraspinous
   Jobert
   olecranon
   patellar
   pituitary
   radial
   retroappendiceal
   Waldeyer
fossa acetabuli
fossa capitelli
fossa hyaloidea
fossa of Treitz
Fourier transformation imaging
Fourier transformation
   zeugmatography
Fourier two-dimensional imaging
Fourier two-dimensional projection
   reconstruction
four-part fracture
four-view chest x-ray
FOV (field of view)
fovea
fovea centralis
fovea inferior
foveola, gastric
fraction
   ejection
   ventricular ejection

fracture
  abduction
  acute
  agenetic
  anatomic
  angulated
  ankle mortise
  apophyseal
  articular
  Atkin epiphyseal
  atrophic
  avulsion
  axial compression
  Barton
  basal neck
  baseball finger
  basilar femoral neck
  bending
  Bennett
  bicondylar
  bimalleolar ankle
  blow-in
  blow-out
  boot-top
  both bone
  boxer's
  bucket-handle
  bumper
  bunk bed
  burst, bursting
  butterfly
  buttonhole
  capillary
  cartwheel
  cementum
  cervicotrochanteric
  chance
  chauffeur
  chevron (V-shaped)
  chip
  chisel
  circumferential

fracture *(cont.)*
  clay shoveler's
  cleavage
  closed
  closed break
  Colles
  comminuted
  comminuted bursting
  comminuted intra-articular
  comminuted teardrop
  complete
  complex
  complicated
  composite
  compound
  compression of cervical vertebral
    body
  compression of thoracic spine
  condylar compression
  condylar split
  congenital
  contrecoup
  cortical
  Cotton ankle
  dashboard
  decompression of
  depressed
  derby hat
  diacondylar
  diaphyseal
  diastatic
  direct
  dishpan
  dislocation
  displaced
  dogleg
  dome
  double
  Dupuytren
  Duverney
  dyscrasic
  en coin

fracture *(cont.)*

endocrine
en rave
epicondylar
epiphyseal slip
Essex-Lopresti calcaneal
extra-articular
extracapsular
fatigue
femoral neck
fissure
four-part
Frykman radial
Galeazzi
Garden femoral neck
Gosselin
greenstick
grenade-thrower's
Guérin
gutter
hairline
hamate tail
hangman's (C2)
healed
hemicondylar
hickory-stick
hockey-stick
horizontal maxillary
humeral head-splitting
impacted
impacted subcapital
impacted valgus
incomplete
indented (of skull)
indirect
inflammatory
infraction
intercondylar
internally fixed
interperiosteal
intertrochanteric
intra-articular

fracture *(cont.)*

intracapsular
intraperiosteal
intrauterine (of fetus)
irreducible
ischioacetabular
Jefferson (of C1)
joint
Jones
Kocher
lateral wedge (of vertebral body)
lead-pipe
Le Fort I; II; III
linear
Lisfranc
local compression
local decompression
long bone
longitudinal
loose
Maisonneuve fibular
Malgaigne pelvic
mallet
malunited
march
midshaft
medial epicondyle
minimally displaced
monomalleolar ankle
Monteggia
Montercaux
Moore
multangular ridge
multiple
navicular
naviculocapitate
neoplastic
neurogenic
neuropathic
nightstick
nonarticular radial head
nondisplaced

fracture *(cont.)*
  oblique
  occult
  old
  olecranon
  one-part
  open
  open-break
  osteochondral
  Pais
  paratrooper
  parry
  patellar
  pathologic
  Pauwels
  pedicle
  pelvic rim
  pelvic ring
  perforating
  periarticular
  peripheral
  peritrochanteric
  phalangeal
  physeal plate
  Piedmont
  pillion
  pillow
  ping-pong
  plateau
  pond
  posterior element
  Pott ankle
  pressure
  pyramidal
  Quervain
  radial head
  resecting
  reverse Barton
  reverse Colles
  ring
  Rolando
  Salter

fracture *(cont.)*
  Salter I-VI
  Salter-Harris type II
  secondary
  segmental
  Segond
  senile subcapital
  SER-IV (supination, external
    rotation-type IV)
  shaft
  shear
  Shepherd
  sideswipe elbow
  silver-fork (Colles)
  simple
  skier's
  Skillern
  Smith
  spiral
  splintered
  split compression
  spontaneous
  sprain
  sprinter's
  stable
  stairstep
  stellate
  stellate skull
  Stieda
  strain
  stress
  subcapital
  subcutaneous
  subperiosteal
  subtrochanteric
  supracondylar femoral
  surgical neck
  T
  T condylar
  T-shaped
  teardrop
  three-part

fracture *(cont.)*
  through-and-through
  tibial plafond
  tibial plateau
  Tillaux
  torsion
  torus
  total condylar depression
  transcapitate
  transcervical femoral
  transcondylar
  transepiphyseal
  transhamate
  transscaphoid
  transtriquetral
  transverse
  transverse maxillary
  trimalleolar ankle
  triplane
  triquetral
  trophic
  tuft
  two-part
  ulnar styloid
  undisplaced
  unilateral
  unstable
  ununited
  V-shaped (chevron)
  vertebral wedge compression
  vertebra plana
  vertical
  vertical shear
  wagon wheel
  Wagstaffe
  wedge
  wedge compression
  wedged
  willow
  Y
  Y-T
fracture at base of odontoid

fracture at waist of odontoid
fracture by contrecoup
fracture classification
fracture-dislocation of forearm,
  Monteggia
fracture en coin
fracture en rave
fracture fragments, union of
fracture injury
fracture nonunion, torsion wedge
fracture of pedicle of axis (C2)
  (hangman's fracture)
fracture within capsule of joint
fracture zone
fragment
  alignment of fracture
  articular
  avulsed fracture
  bone
  butterfly fracture
  chondral
  cortical
  disk
  displaced
  fracture
  free
  free-floating cartilaginous
  loose
  major fracture
  osteochondral
  smear
free air in diaphragm
free fluid
free fragment
free induction decay (FID)
free-floating cartilaginous fragment
free pleural effusion
Freiberg disease
Freiberg infraction
French catheter
French draining catheter
French introducer catheter

French pigtail catheter
French shaft balloon
frequency, Larmor
frequency-related peak
friable mucosa
Friedreich foot
frogleg view
frontal bone
frontal horn
frontal lobe
frontal plane
frontal sinus
frontal suture
frontal view
frontoparietal
frothy colonic mucosa
Frykman radial fracture
full bladder technique
full column barium enema
function, swallowing
functional disorder
functional disturbance
fundal

fundus
   bald gastric
   gallbladder
   gastric
fundus uteri
fungating
funiculus cuneatus
funiculus dorsalis
funiculus gracilis
funiculus medullae spinalis
funiculus ventralis
funnel chest
funnel deformity
funnel pelvis
funny bone
fusiform dilatation
fusiform widening of duct
fusion
   calcaneotibial
   diaphyseal-epiphyseal
   joint
   spinal

# G, g

Ga–67 (gallium citrate) isotope
Galeazzi fracture of radius
gallbladder
   bilobed
   chronically inflamed
   Courvoisier
   dilated
   edematous
   fish-scale
   floating
   folded fundus
   fundal portion of
   hourglass
   inflamed
   mobile
   multiseptate
   porcelain
   stasis
   strawberry
   thick-walled
   thin-walled
   wandering
gallbladder bed
gallbladder calculus
gallbladder hydrops
gallbladder polyp
gallbladder stasis
gallbladder ultrasound
gallium scan
gallium-67 citrate imaging
gallstone
   radiolucent
   silent
gallstone migration
gamekeeper's thumb
gamma camera
Gamna-Gandy body
Gamna-Gandy nodule

Gamna nodule
Gamna disease
Gandy-Nanta disease
ganglia, basal
ganglioneuroma
Ganser diverticulum
gantry of lithotripsy machine
gantry tilt
Garden femoral neck fracture
Garré disease
Gartner duct
gas
   abdominal
   bowel
   coursing of
   small-bowel
gas density line
gaseous distention
gas-forming organism in bowel wall
gas in soft tissues
gas pattern
gastrectomy
gastric air bubble
gastric antrum
gastric channel
gastric catarrh
gastric distention
gastric fistula
gastric foveola
gastric fundus, bald
gastric impression on liver
gastric mucosal pattern
gastric outline
gastric partition
gastric pull-through segment
gastric reflux
gastric remnant
gastric ulcer

gastric window
gastritis
   acute erosive (AEG)
   alkaline reflux
   antral
   atrophic
   bile reflux
   emphysematous
   erosive
   giant hypertrophic
   granulomatous
   nonerosive nonspecific
   polypous
   proliferative hypertrophic
   pseudomembranous
   reflux bile
   stress
   ulcerative
   varioliform
   zonal
gastrocnemius muscle
gastroenteritis
gastroenterocolitis
gastroenterostomy
gastroesophageal incompetence
gastroesophageal junction
gastroesophageal reflux (GER)
gastroesophageal variceal plexus
gastrogastrostomy
Gastrografin contrast medium
gastrointestinal (GI) tract
gastrojejunal
gastroptosis
gastroscopy
gastrostomy, Beck
gastrotomy
Gastrovist contrast medium
gated blood (pool) cardiac wall
   motion study
gated blood pool ventriculogram
gated cardiac blood pool imaging
gated equilibrium blood pool
   scanning

gated view
gating, cardiac
gauge
gauss
gaussian distribution
gaussian line saturation
gaussian mode profile laser beam
Gaynor-Hart position
Gd-DTPA radioisotope
GE 8800 CT scanner
GE 9800 high-resolution CT
   scanner
Gee-Herter disease
gemellary pregnancy
generator, Van de Graaff
genial tubercle of mandible
geniculate
geniculum
genu extrorsum
genu impressum
genu introrsum
genu of pancreatic duct
genu recurvatum
genu valgum
genu varum
geometry factor
GER (gastroesophageal reflux)
GERD (gastroesophageal reflux
   disease)
Gerdy tubercle
geriatric features on chest x-ray
gestation
   extrauterine
   intrauterine
gestational age
Ghon complex
Ghon primary lesion
Ghon tubercle
GI (gastrointestinal)
giardiasis
gibbous deformity
gibbus (n.); gibbous (adj.)

girdle, pelvic
glabella
gland
   adrenal
   hilar
   lymph
   parotid
   pineal
   pituitary
   suprarenal
   thymus
   thyroid
glandular tissue
Glénard disease
glenohumeral joint dislocation
glenoid fossa
glenoid process
Glidewire, Radiofocus
glioblastoma
glioma, butterfly-type
gliosis
Glisson capsule
globe, optic
globular
globus hystericus
glomerular
glottis
glucagon
gluteal region
gluteus maximus
gluteus muscle
gm (gram)
goiter, substernal
Golay coil
GoLytely bowel prep
gonarthritis
gonial angle (of mandible)
Goodpasture syndrome
gooseneck deformity of outflow
   tract
Gosselin fracture
gout, tophaceous

graafian follicle
graafian vesicle
gradient
   pressure
   rephasing
gradient coil
gradient echo sequence
gradient magnetic field
graft, vascular
gram (gm)
Granger view
granuloma (pl. granulomata)
granulomatous disease
granulomatous gastritis
Graser diverticulum
GRASS (gradient recalled acquisition in a steady state)
Gratiolet convolutions
gravid uterus
gravida
gray (Gy)
gray matter
gray-scale imaging
gray-scale ultrasound
greater curvature of stomach
greater multangular bone
greater sciatic notch
greater trochanter
greater tuberosity
great vessels, transposition of
greenstick fracture
grenade thrower's fracture
grenz ray
Greulich and Pyle (bone age scale)
Grollman pigtail catheter
groove defect of humeral head
groove, sagittal
Groshong catheter
ground-glass appearance
ground-glass opacity
ground state
growth plate

Gruber fossa
Gruentzig (Grüntzig) catheter
Guérin fracture
guide wire
    Bentson
    J-curve movable core
    Lunderquist exchange
    Lunderquist-Ring torque
    Newton
Gull disease
gumma (pl. gummas or gummata)
gummas of ribs

gun, Bard bioptic
gun stock deformity
gutter fracture
Gy (gray)
gynecoid pelvis
gyriform calcification
gyromagnetic ratio
Gyroscan, Philips
gyrus
gyrus cinguli
gyrus fornicatus
gyrus hippocampi

# H, h

H–1–H (headhunter) catheter
H/S catheter (hysterosalpingog-
    raphy)
habenula
habitual dislocation
Haeckerman area
Haglund deformity
Haglund disease
Hagner disease
hairline fracture
half-life
    antibody
    biological
    effective
hallux flexus deformity
hallux malleus deformity
hallux rigidus deformity
hallux valgus deformity
hallus varus deformity
halo effect
hamartoma
    duodenal wall
    pancreatic
hamartomatous lesion

hamartomatous polyp
hamate bone
hamate tail fracture
hamatum
hammertoe
Hampton hump
Hampton line
hamstring muscle
hamstring tendon
hamulus
hand injection of contrast medium
Hand-Schüller-Christian disease
hangman's fracture
Harrington distraction system
Harrison sulcus
Hartmann point
Hashimoto disease
Hashimoto thyroiditis
Haudek niche
haustral blunting
haustral fold
haustral indentation
haustral markings
haustral pattern

haustral pouch
haustrations
haustrum (pl. haustra)
haversian canal
Hawkins breast localization needle
    with FlexStrand cable
hazy infiltrates
head
  femoral
  humeral
  long
  metatarsal
  radial
  short
head of barium column
head of femur
head of humerus
head of pancreas
head of radius
headhunter catheter
heart
  athletic
  balloon-shaped
  beer
  boat-shaped
  boot-shaped
  cervical
  crisscross
  enlarged
  fatty
  fibroid
  flask-shaped
  frosted
  hanging (suspended)
  horizontal
  hypoplastic
  pear-shaped
  pendulous
  Quain fatty
  round
  sabot
  semihorizontal

heart *(cont.)*
  semivertical
  snowman
  suspended
  teardrop
  vertical
  wooden shoe
Heberden disease
Heberden nodes
Hedspa
heel bone
heel, Sorbol
heel tendon
Heister valves
Helmholtz coil
Helmholtz configuration
hemal arch
hemangioma
hemarthrosis
hematochezia
hematogenous
hematoma
  evolving
  intracranial
  retromembranous
  subdural
hematomediastinum (hemomediastinum)
hematopericardium (hemopericardium)
hematuria
hemiatrophy
hemicolectomy
hemidiaphragm, hemidiaphragmatic
hemisphere, cerebral
hemithorax
hemodynamic assessment
hemodynamic reserve impairment
hemoglobinopathy
hemomediastinum (hemato-
  mediastinum)
hemopericardium (hematopericardium)

hemoptysis
hemorrhage
hemorrhagic cyst
hemosiderosis
hemothorax
Henderson-Jones disease
Henke trigone
Henle, jejunal interposition of
Henle loop
Henle sheath
Henoch purpura
Hensing fold
heparin
heparinized blood
hepatic angiography
hepatic arteriogram
hepatic bed
hepatic cyst
hepatic diverticulum
hepatic ductal system
hepatic duct bifurcation
hepatic flexure of colon
hepatic insufficiency
hepatic venous outflow
hepatic venous web disease
hepatic web dilation
hepatization
hepatobiliary scan
hepatojugular reflux
Hepatolite
hepatolithiasis
hepatoma
hepatomalacia
hepatomegaly
hepatoptosis
hepatosplenomegaly
hereditary
hernia
    abdominal wall
    axial hiatal
    Bochdalek
    cecal

hernia *(cont.)*
    congenital
    diaphragmatic
    direct
    epigastric
    femoral
    hiatal
    hiatus
    incarcerated
    indirect
    inguinal
    Littre
    obturator
    paraesophageal hiatal
    paraileostomal
    Richter
    Rieux
    rolling hiatal
    scrotal
    sliding
    sliding-type
    sliding-type hiatal
    strangulated
    Treitz
    umbilical
    ventral
hernia defect
hernia pouch
hernia sac
herniated disk
herniated nucleus pulposus
heterogeneous uptake
heterotopic pancreas
heterotopic pregnancy
Hexabrix contrast medium
hexadactyly
Hey amputation
hiatal hernia (see *hernia)*
hiatus
    adductor
    esophageal

hiatus hernia
Hickman catheter
hickory-stick fracture
Hieshima coaxial catheter
high-contrast film
high-density linear array
high field strength scanner
high-grade stenosis
high resolution coronal cuts on
    CT scan
high-riding patella (patella alta)
hilar dance
hilar gland enlargement
hilar haze
hilar lymph node
hilar mass
hilar node
hilar reaction
Hill-Sachs deformity
Hilton law
hilum (pl. hila)
hilus (pl. hili)
hilus of kidney
hilus of lung
hindfoot
hinge joint
hip bone (os coxae)
hippocampal
hippocampus
Hippuran contrast medium
Hirschsprung disease
His band
His bundle
His spindle
histiocytosis X
histology, histologic
histoplasmoma
histoplasmosis
Hitachi ultrasound
Hodgkin disease
Hodgson disease
Hoffa disease

Hoffmann atrophy
holosystolic
Holter monitor
Holt-Oram syndrome
Holzknecht stomach
homalocephalous
Homer Mammalok hook wire
homogeneity
homogeneous
homogeneous acinar consolidation
homogeneous echo pattern
honeycomb lung
honeycomb pattern
horizontal lie
horizontal maxillary fracture
horizontal plane
horn, frontal
horseshoe appearance
horseshoe configuration
horseshoe kidney
hose-pipe appearance of terminal
    ileum
hot nodule
Hounsfield unit (on CT scan)
hourglass bladder
hourglass constriction of
    gallbladder
hourglass stomach
housemaid's knee
HSG (hysterosalpingography)
Hughston view
humeral bone
humeral head
humeral head-splitting fracture
humeroradial articulation
humeroulnar articulation
humerus
hump
    buffalo
    dowager's
    Hampton
Huppert disease

hyaline membrane disease
hyaloid fossa
hydatidiform mole
hydramnios
hydrocele
hydrocephalic
hydrocephalus, hydrocephalous
hydrogen proton imaging
hydronephrosis
hydropericardium
hydroperitoneum
hydropneumothorax
hydrops of gallbladder
hydrosalpinx
hyoid bone
Hypaque contrast medium
Hypaque-Cysto contrast medium
Hypaque-M contrast medium
Hypaque Meglumine contrast
    medium
Hypaque Sodium contrast medium
hyperaeration
hyperconcentration of contrast
    medium
hyperdense
hyperechoic area
hyperextension injury
hyperinflation, pulmonary
hyperintense mass
hyperintensity
hypermotility
hyperostosis
    ankylosing spinal
    diffuse idiopathic sclerosis
        (DISH)
    infantile cortical
hyperostosis corticalis deformans
    juvenilis
hyperostosis corticalis generalisata
hyperostosis cranii
hyperostosis frontalis interna
hyperostosis of anterolateral
    vertebral column

hyperostosis of spine, senile
    ankylosing
hyperperistalsis
hyperplasia
    adenomatous
    ductal
hyperplastic
hyperprochoresis
hyperpronation
hyperrugosity
hypersthenia
hypersthenic
hypertelorism
hypertension, pulmonary artery
hypertensive
hypertonic
hypertonicity
hypertrophic arthritis
hypertrophic gastropathy
hypertrophic marginal spurring
hypertrophic pulmonary osteo-
    arthropathy
hypertrophic spurring
hypertrophy
    left ventricular (LVH)
    pyloric
    right ventricular (RVH)
hypertrophy of bone
hypoaeration
hypodense area
hypodense lesion
hypoechoic area
hypogammaglobulinemia
hypokinesis, hypokinetic
hypoperistalsis
hypopharyngeal diverticulum
hypopharynx
hypoplasia, bile duct
hypoproteinemia
hypospadias
hypostatic pneumonia
hyposthenia

hyposthenic
hypothalamus
hypothenar eminence
hypotonic duodenography
hystericus, globus

hysterogram
hysterosalpingogram
hysterosalpingography
hysterotubogram

# I, i

$^{131}$I (iodine 131)
IABP (intra-aortic balloon
  pumping)
IBD (inflammatory bowel disease)
IBS (irritable bowel syndrome)
ICS (intercostal space)
IDD (intraluminal duodenal diverticulum)
idiopathic disease
idiopathic intestinal pseudo-
  obstruction
idiopathic megacolon
IDIS (intraoperative digital
  subtraction angiography)
ileitis, regional
ileocecal fat pad
ileocecal junction
ileocecal region
ileocecal valve
  competent
  incompetent
ileocolic fold
ileocolitis
ileogram
ileostogram (loopogram)
ileum, terminal
ileus
  adynamic
  dynamic
  gallstone
  mechanical

ileus *(cont.)*
  meconium
  occlusive
  paralytic
  postoperative
  spastic
Ilfeld-Holder deformity
iliac adenopathy
iliac bone
iliac crest
iliac disease
iliac fossa
iliac lesion
iliac spine
iliac tuberosity
iliofemoral
iliopectineal eminence
iliopsoas muscle
iliopsoas ring
ilium
ill-defined
image
  color-coded
  coronal
  delayed
  multi-echo
  multi-echo coronal
  proton density
  real-time
  scout
  spin-echo

image *(cont.)*
  static
  T1 weighted
  T1 weighted coronal
  T1 weighted sagittal
  T2 weighted
  two-dimensional (2-D)
image acquisition time
imaged (verb)
image intensifier
imaging
  Aloka color Doppler real-time
    2-D blood flow imaging with
    Cine Memory
  antifibrin antibody
  axial
  blood flow
  bone
  contiguous
  echo planar
  gallium-67 citrate
  gray-scale
  hydrogen proton
  ImmuRAID (CEA Tc 99m)
  line
  magnetic resonance (MRI)
  noninvasive
  nuclear bone
  phase
  planar spin
  point
  Purkinje
  sagittal
  sequential plane
  sequential point
  simultaneous volume
  spin-echo
  technetium 99m particle
  three-dimensional Fourier
    transform
  two-dimensional Fourier
    transform
  volume

Imatron C-100 ultrafast CT scanner
IMED intravenous infusion device
immunoblastic
impacted fracture
impacted subcapital fracture
impacted valgus fracture
impedance plethysmography (IPG)
imperforate
impinge, impinging, impingement
improvement, interval
impulse, apical
inanition
incarcerated hernia
incarceration
incarial bone
incisura acetabuli
incisura angularis
incisura clavicularis
incisura costales sterni
incisura fibularis
incisura ischiadica major
incisura radialis
incisura scapulae
incisura semilunaris
incisura ulnaris
incomplete dislocation
incomplete fracture of bone
increased echo signal on ultrasound
increased tracer uptake
incus bone
indented fracture of skull
indirect fracture
indirect hernia
indium 111 labeled leukocyte scan
inelastic collision
infantile cortical hyperostosis
infarct
  bone
  white matter
infarction
  myocardial
  pulmonary

infection, infectious
inferior vena cava
inferiormost
inferior pubic ramus (pl. rami)
infiltrate
   active
   alveolar
   circumscribed
   confluent
   fibronodular
   hazy
   interstitial
   linear
   lung base
   patchy
   peribronchial
   perihilar
   perivascular
   pneumonic
   pulmonary
   reticular
   strandy
infiltration, fatty
infiltration pattern
inflammation of calcaneal bursa
inflammatory bowel disease (IBD)
inflammatory disease
inflammatory fracture
inflammatory process
inflation, air
infraclavicular
infraction, Freiberg
infraglenoid tuberosity
infrapatellar
infrascapular
infraspinous fossa
infundibulum, cerebral
Infuse-a-port catheter
inguinal adenopathy
inguinal hernia
inguinal node
inguinal region

inguinal trigone
inhalation study
inhomogeneity
inhomogeneous echo pattern
inhomogeneous image
inhomogeneous tracer distribution
initial delay in appearance time of
   contrast material
initiate, initiation
injection
   barium (through colostomy)
   hand (done by hand)
   machine (done by machine)
injection of contrast medium
injury
   axial compression (of spine)
   brachial plexus
   contrecoup
   crush
   degloving
   extension (of spine)
   flexion (of spine)
   flexion-distraction (of spine)
   flexion-rotation (of spine)
   hyperextension
   lateral bending (of spine)
   meniscal
   seat belt
   soft tissue
   softball sliding
   traumatic
inlet, pelvic
innominate aneurysm
innominate bone
innominate vein
insertion
in situ
inspiratory effort
inspissated
inspissation of feces
instability
   anterolateral rotary knee

instability *(cont.)*
  dorsal intercalary segment (DISI)
  joint
  rotational
installation
instep
instillation
insufficiency
  aortic
  cardiac
  coronary
  gastric
  hepatic
  ileocecal
  muscular
  myocardial
  parathyroid
  pulmonary
  pyloric
  renal
  thyroid
  tricuspid
  uterine
  velopharyngeal
  venous
  vertebrobasilar
insufflation, tubal
integrity and alignment
intensity
  low signal
  signal
interarticularis
interatrial septum
intercarpal articulation
interclavicular notch
intercondylar eminence
intercondylar fracture
intercondylar notch
intercondyloid eminence
intercondyloid fossa
intercondyloid notch
intercostal space (ICS)

intercristal diameter
interface, acoustic
intergluteal cleft
interlaminar
interlobar septum
intermaxillary spine
intermetacarpal articulation
intermetatarsal angle
intermittent diffuse esophageal
  spasm
internal capsule
internal carotid system
internal conjugate diameter
internal iliac artery
internal-external drainage catheter
internal tibial torsion (ITT)
interosseous membrane
interosseous space
interparietal bone
interpediculate
interperiosteal fracture
interphalangeal articulation
interposition, soft tissue
interpulse time
intersigmoid recess
interspace, disk
intersperse
interspinous pseudarthrosis
interstices, bone
interstitial changes
interstitial edema
interstitial fibrosis
interstitial fluid
interstitial infiltrate
interstitial marking
interstitial meniscal tear
interstitial prominence
interstitial shadowing
intertarsal
intertrochanteric plate
intertubercular diameter
interval change

interval improvement
interval progression
interval resolution
interventional radiography
interventricular septal defect
interventricular septum
intervertebral disk
intervertebral disk narrowing
intervertebral foramen
intestinal atresia
intestinal diverticulum
intestinal follicle
intestinal infantilism
intestinal villous architecture
intestinal web
intestine, blind
intimal remodeling
intra-abdominal fat
intra-acetabular
intra-aneurysmal thrombus
intra-aortic balloon pumping
  (IABP)
intra-articular fracture
intra-articular loose body
intracapsular fracture
intrachondrial bone
intracortical osteogenic sarcoma
intracranial
intractable ulcer
intraesophageal stent
intrahepatic atresia (IHA)
intrahepatic biliary drainage
  catheter
intrahepatic biliary radicles, dilated
intrahepatic biliary tract dilatation
intrahepatic biliary tree
intraluminal duodenal diverticulum
  (IDD)
intraluminal mass
intramammary
intramedullary fixation
intramural air in colon

intramural diverticulum
intramural thrombus
intraoperative digital subtraction
  (IDIS) angiography
intraoperative pancreatography
intraosseous venography
intraosseous wiring
intraparenchymal
intraperiosteal fracture
intraperitoneal air
intraperitoneal fluid
intraperitoneal rupture
intrapulmonary
intrarenal
intrathecal imaging
intrathoracic dislocation of shoulder
intrathoracic stomach
intrathoracic thyroid
intratracheal
intrauterine fracture (of fetus)
intrauterine pregnancy
intravenous (I.V.)
intravenous bolus injection of
  contrast medium
intravenous cholangiography (IVC)
intravenous pyelogram (IVP)
intravenous urography
intraventricular
intrinsic minus deformity
  (clawhand)
intrinsic minus hallux
intrinsic plus deformity
introducer
  Bentson
  Desilets-Hoffman
  Schwartz
introitus
Intropaque contrast medium
intubation
intussusception
  bowel
  retrograde

intussuscipiens
invagination of ligament into joint
invasive
inversion recovery image
inversion recovery sequence
inversion recovery technique
inversion time (TI)
inversus, situs
inverted V sign
in vivo method
in vivo technique
involucrum
iocetamic acid contrast medium
iodamine meglumine contrast
　　medium
iodinated contrast medium
iodine 131 ($^{131}$I)
iodine 131 MIBG scintigraphy
iodine, sodium
iodipamide meglumine contrast
　　medium
iodized oil
iohexol
ion exchange
ionization chamber
Iopamidol
iopanoic acid contrast medium
iopentol nonionic contrast medium
iophendylate contrast medium
iopydone contrast medium
iothalamate
ioversol contrast medium
ioxaglate meglumine contrast
　　medium
ioxaglate sodium contrast medium
IPG (impedance plethysmography)
ipodate calcium contrast medium

ipsilateral
irreducible dislocation
irregular bone
irregularity
irritable bowel syndrome (IBS)
irritable colon
ischemia
ischial bone
ischial spine
ischial tuberosity
ischioacetabular fracture
island
　　bone
　　bony
　　mucosal
isodense
isodensity
isolated dislocation of semilunar
　　bone
Isopaque contrast medium
isosulfan blue contrast medium
isotope (see radioisotope)
isotope scan
isotope, stable
isotope venogram
isotopic skeletal survey
isotropic 3-D or volume study
Isovue-300 contrast medium
Isovue-370 contrast medium
Isovue-M 200 contrast medium
Isovue-M 300 contrast medium
ITT (internal tibial torsion)
I.V. (intravenous)
Ivalon sponge
IVC (intravenous cholangiography)
ivory bone
IVP (intravenous pyelogram)

# J, j

JB1 catheter
JB3 catheter
J-curve movable core guide wire
Jackson membrane
Jaffe-Lichtenstein disease
Jansen disease
jaundice
jaw bone
Jefferson fracture of atlas
jejunal loop interposition of Henle
jejunum
Jelco catheter
Jewett nail
Jobert fossa
joint
    AC (acromioclavicular)
    atlantoaxial
    ball-and-socket
    calcaneocuboid
    carpometacarpal
    Charcot
    Chopart
    condyloid
    costovertebral
    cuneiform
    DIP (distal interphalangeal)
    distal interphalangeal (DIP)
    ellipsoid
    facet
    flail
    free knee
    glenohumeral
    gliding
    hinge
    hip capsule
    immovable
    Lisfranc
    Luschka

joint *(cont.)*
    metacarpal-phalangeal (MCP)
    metacarpophalangeal (MCP)
    metatarsal-phalangeal (MTP)
    metatarsocuneiform
    metatarsophalangeal (MTP)
    mortise
    PIP (proximal interphalangeal)
    pisotriquetral
    pivot
    saddle
    SI (sacroiliac)
    sternoclavicular
    subtalar
    synovial
    talonavicular
    tarsal-metatarsal
    tarsometatarsal
    temporomandibular
    tibiofibular
    tibiotalar
    uncovertebral
    weightbearing
joint capsule
joint congruity
joint, facet
joint fracture
joint incongruity
joint of Luschka
joint space
    cartilage
    metatarsal-phalangeal
    patellofemoral
    subtalar
    tarsal-metatarsal
    tibial-talar
joint space narrowing
joint swelling

Jones fracture
Judkins technique of selective
  coronary arteriography
jugular catheter
jugular vein
jugulodigastric chain
jugulodigastric node
junction
  anorectal
  cardioesophageal (CE)
  choledochopancreatic ductal
  cystic-choledochal
  duodenojejunal
  esophagogastric (EG)
  fundic-antral

junction *(cont.)*
  gastroesophageal (GE)
  ileocecal
  meniscosynovial
  pancreaticobiliary ductal
  pelviureteral
  pyloroduodenal
  tracheoesophageal (TE)
  ureteropelvic
juvenile Paget disease
juxta-articular
juxta-articulation
juxtacortical chondroma
juxtapapillary diverticulum
juxtapyloric ulcer

# K, k

k-capture
Kahler disease
Keith node
Kent-His bundle
Kerckring fold
Kerley A line
Kerley B line
Kerley C line
Kernohan notch
keV or kev (kiloelectron volt)
kHz (kilohertz)
kidney, kidneys
  abdominal
  arteriosclerotic
  atrophic
  cicatricial
  congenital absence of
  congested
  contracted
  cortical scarring of
  crush

kidney *(cont.)*
  cyanotic
  cystic
  disk of
  distended
  double
  doughnut
  duplication of left
  duplication of right
  dysfunctional
  ectopic
  edematous
  fatty
  fibrotic
  floating
  Formad
  fused
  Goldblatt
  granular
  hilum of
  hilus of

kidney *(cont.)*
  horseshoe
  hypermobile
  infundibulum of
  irregular
  lobe of
  lobulated
  long axis of
  lumbar
  medullary sponge
  movable
  mural
  myeloma
  nonfunctioning
  pelvic
  pelvis of
  polycystic
  porous
  ptosis of
  ptotic
  Rose-Bradford
  sacciform
  scarred
  sclerotic
  shriveled
  sigmoid
  sponge
  spongy
  supernumerary
  suspension of
  thoracic
  tomography of both
  wandering
kidney scan
kidney shadow
kidney stone, passing of
kidneys, ureters, and bladder (KUB)
kidney transplant
Kienböck disease
Kienböck dislocation
Kiernan spaces in liver
Kilian line

Kilian pelvis
kiloelectron volt (keV or kev)
kilohertz (kHz)
kinetic energy
kinetic gallbladder study
Kinevac contrast medium
kink in bowel
kink in intestine
kink, Lane
Kirchner diverticulum
Klatzkin tumor
Klippel-Feil syndrome
knee
  anterior cruciate deficit of
  Brodie
  dislocated
  housemaid's
  locked
kneecap
knee-like bend in a structure
knob, aortic
knobby process
knuckle bone
knuckle of colon
Kocher fracture
Köhler disease
Köhler-Pellegrini-Stieda disease
Köhler tarsal scaphoiditis
Kohlrausch fold
Kölliker nucleus
Kopans needle
krypton
KUB (kidneys, ureters, and urinary
  bladder)
Kugelberg-Welander disease
Kulchitsky cells
Kümmell disease
kyllosis
kymography
kyphoscoliosis
kyphosis, kyphotic

# L, l

L (lumbar vertebra)
L1–L5 (five lumbar vertebrae)
L5–S1 vertebral interspace
LS (lumbosacral) spine
Labbe triangle
labeling, radioisotope
labia (pl. of labium)
labial
labium (pl. labia)
lacertus fibrosus
laciniate ligament
lacrimal bone
lacuna cerebri
lacunae (pl. of lacuna)
Laennec cirrhosis
lambdoid suture
lamellated bone
lamina cribrosa
lamina papyracea
laminated calculus
laminectomy
laminography
Lane band
Lane disease
Lane kink
Langenbeck triangle
LAO (left anterior oblique) position
Larmor equation
Larmor frequency
Larmor precession
Larsen disease
Larsen-Johansson disease
laryngocele
larynx, laryngeal
laser printer, Ektascan
last menstrual period (LMP)
late film
lateral abdominal aortogram

lateral bending injury (of spine)
lateral cervical spine film
lateral condyle
lateral decubitus view
lateral position
lateral projection, view
lateral reflection of colon
lateral sclerosis
lateral tomography
lateral ventricle
lateral wedge fracture of vertebral
    body
lateroconal fascia
lattice relaxation time
lattice vibrations
law, Hilton
Law view
layering of gallstones
lead-pipe colon
lead-pipe fracture
leaf of diaphragm
leakage of contrast medium
leather bottle stomach
leaves of diaphragm
Le Fort amputation
Le Fort I apertognathia repair
Le Fort I fracture
Le Fort II fracture
Le Fort II pyramidal fracture of
    maxilla
Le Fort III fracture
left anterior oblique (LAO) position
left posterior oblique (LPO)
    position
left ventricular ejection fraction
left ventricular hypertrophy (LVH)
left-to-right shift

leg
  baker
  bayonet
Legg disease
Legg-Calvé disease
Legg-Calvé-Perthes disease
Legg-Perthes disease
Legg-Calvé-Waldenström disease
leiomyoma
leiomyosarcoma
Leksell stereotaxic device
lemostenosis
lenticular bone of hand
Lenzmann point
Lenz point
leptomeningeal cyst
lesion
  adrenal
  annular
  apical
  apple core
  atheromatous
  calcified
  cavitary
  circular
  circumscribed
  coin
  cold
  constricting esophageal
  cortical
  desiccated
  destructive
  discrete
  doughnut
  dumbbell
  echogenic
  ellipsoid
  esophageal
  extrinsic
  focal
  fungating mass
  Ghon

lesion *(cont.)*
  granular
  gross
  high-density
  hot
  intramedullary
  intrinsic
  invasive
  left lower lobe (LLL)
  left upper lobe (LUL)
  lipomatous
  localized
  low-density
  lytic (osteolytic)
  lytic bone
  malignant
  mass
  metastatic bone
  napkin ring
  neoplastic
  nevoid
  nodular
  noninvasive
  obstructive
  occlusive
  occult
  osseous
  osteoblastic
  outcropping of
  pedunculated
  periapical
  photon-deficient
  plaquelike
  polypoid
  pontine
  primary
  pulmonary
  questionable
  radiographic
  radiographic stability of
  radiopaque
  rectal

lesion *(cont.)*
    rectosigmoid polypoid
    recurrent
    resectable
    rib
    right lower lobe (RLL)
    right upper lobe (RUL)
    satellite
    scirrhous
    sessile
    sharply demarcated circum-
        ferential
    slowly developing
    solitary
    sonolucent
    space-occupying
    spontaneous
    suspicious
    target
    temporal lobe
    tongue
    total
    tuberculous
    ulcerated
    ulcerating
    ulcerative
    undifferentiated
    unresectable
    vascular
    wedge-shaped
    wide field
lesser curvature of stomach
lesser multangular bone
lesser omentum
lesser sciatic notch
lesser trochanter
leukemia
level
    air-fluid
    fluid
levoscoliosis
LFV (large field of view)
lidocaine

lie
    horizontal
    longitudinal
    transverse
Lieberkühn crypt
lienography
LiF (lithium fluoride)
ligament
    acromiocoracoid
    adipose
    arcuate
    Bardinet
    Barkow
    Brodie
    calcaneoclavicular
    Caldani
    cruciate
    cruciatum cruris
    iliopubic
    laciniate
    Poupart
    rhomboid
    stellate
    Weitbrecht
ligamenta (pl. of ligamentum)
ligamenta cruciata digitorum pedis
ligamenta cruciata genu
ligamenta patellae
ligamenta tarsi dorsalia
ligamentum annulare radii
ligamentum collaterale ulnare
ligamentum coracoacromiale
ligamentum coracoclaviculare
ligamentum coracohumerale
ligamentum cuboideonaviculare
    dorsale
ligamentum deltoideum
ligamentum flavum
ligamentum nuchae
ligamentum plantare longum
ligamentum sternoclaviculare
ligamentum teres
ligamentum trapezoideum

ligamentous disruption
limited film; view
line, lines
   anterior junction
   arterial
   central venous pressure (CVP)
   costophrenic septal
   dentate
   fat
   gas density
   Hampton
   iliopectineal
   Kerley A
   Kerley B
   Kerley C
   Kilian
   Lorentzian
   low-intensity
   midaxillary
   pectinate
   popliteal
   pubococcygeal
   Retzius
   skin
   subcutaneous fat
   suture
   Z
linea intertrochanterica
linear accelerator, Mitsubishi
linear amplifier
linear array
   Acuson 5 MHz
   convex
   high-density
linear band of maximal radiolucency
linear density of bone
linear fracture
linear infiltrate
linear interstitial density
linear opacity
linear phased arrays
linear scanning

linear streak
linear tomography
line imaging
line of Retzius
line saturation
   gaussian
   Lorentzian
line scanning
line width
liquid crystal thermogram
lingual bone
lingula
lingula pulmonis
lingular nodule
linitis plastica
lip, posterior
Lipiodol contrast medium
lipoid pneumonia
lipoma
liponecrosis
Liquipake contrast medium
Lisfranc dislocation
Lissauer column
lithiasis, renal (also renolithiasis)
Lithostar machine
Littre hernia
Litzmann obliquity
liver
   cirrhotic
   enlarged
   fatty
   nodular
   noncirrhotic
   nutmeg
   polycystic
   polylobar
   prominent
   shrunken
   wandering
liver bed
liver edge
liver, kidneys, and spleen (LKS)

liver parenchyma, normal
liver scan, radionuclide
liver scintiphotograph
liver span
liver-spleen scan
Livingston triangle
LKS (liver, kidneys, and spleen)
LMP (last menstrual period)
lobar
lobe
    azygos
    caudate
    collapsed
    frontal
    lower
    middle
    occipital
    parietal
    pyramidal
    quadrate
    Riedel
    temporal
    thyroid
    upper
lobular architecture of liver
lobule
local compression fracture
local decompression of fracture
localization grid
loculated effusion
Loeffler syndrome
Lohlein diameter
long bone
long bone fracture
long head
long TR/TE ($T_2$ weighted image)
longitudinal fissure
longitudinal fracture
longitudinal lie
longitudinal taenia musculature
longitudinal ultrasonic biometry

loop
    afferent
    air-filled
    bowel
    colonic
    contiguous
    duodenal
    efferent
    intestinal
    jejunal
    N-shaped sigmoid
    sentinel
    sigmoid
    small-bowel
    transverse colon
loop of bowel
loop of Henle
loopogram (ileostogram)
loops of bowel, dilated
loose fracture
Looser-Milkman syndrome
Lorad M-II D mammographic
    system
lordosis
    cervical
    lumbar
    reversal of
    thoracic
lordotic curve
lordotic position; view
Lorentzian line saturation
loss of sigmoid curve
Louis angle
Low-Beers projection; view
low-contrast film
low-contrast structure
low-density lesion
low-dose film mammographic
    technique
low-dose mammography
low-intensity line
lower lung field

lower pole of kidney
lower pole of patella
lower pulmonary artery
low signal intensity
LPO (left posterior oblique)
    position
lucency, interspersed
lucent defect
Ludwig angle
lumbar artery
lumbarization
lumbar scoliosis
lumbar spine
lumbar transverse process
lumbar vertebra
lumbosacral kyphosis
lumbosacral series
lumbosacral spine
lumen
    attenuated
    clot-filled
    occluded
    patent
lumina (pl. of lumen)
luminal narrowing
lunate bone
lunate dislocation
lunatomalacia
Lunderquist exchange guide wire
Lunderquist-Ring torque guide wire
lung
    atelectatic
    collapsed
    expanded
    root of
    well-inflated
lung base
lung field
lung/heart activity ratio
lung/heart ratio of thallium 201
    activity

lung markings
lung scan
lung zone
Luschka crypts of gallbladder
    mucosa
Luschka, joint of
Lutembacher syndrome
luxated bone
luxatio coxae congenita
luxatio erecta shoulder dislocation
luxatio imperfecta
luxatio perinealis
luxation
LVH (left ventricular hypertrophy)
lymphadenopathy
    hilar
    mediastinal
lymphangiectasia, congenital
    dislocation
lymphangiographic contrast
lymphangiography
lymphangitic carcinomatosis
lymphangitic metastasis
lymphatic cachexia
Lymphazurin (isosulfan blue)
lymph gland
lymph node, hilar
lymphoblastoma
lymphocele
lymphoma
    Burkitt
    granulomatous
    infiltrative
    nodular
    polypoid
    ulcerative
lymphosarcoma
lytic area
lytic bone lesion
lytic change
lytic (osteolytic) lesion

# M, m

Mackenzie point
MacLean-Maxwell disease
macrocephaly
macrocolon
Magendie, foramen of
magnetic dipole
magnetic resonance imaging (MRI)
magnetic resonance spectroscopy
    (MRS)
magnetogyric ratio
Magnetom SP MRI imager
Magnevist contrast medium
main stem bronchus
Maisonneuve fibular fracture
malalignment
malangulation
malar bone
Malecot catheter
malformation
    anorectal
    arteriovenous (AVM)
    Chiari II
Malgaigne fracture
malignancy
malignant nephrosclerosis
malleolar
malleoli (pl. of malleolus)
malleolus
    lateral
    medial
malleolus fibulae
malleolus tibiae
mallet, bone
mallet finger
Mallinckrodt catheter
malpighian vesicle
malrotation
malposition

malrotation of intestine
malum coxae senilis
malum perforans pedis
malunion of fracture fragments
malunited
mammectomy
Mamex DC mammography
mammalation
mammogram
    microfocal spot
    screen-film
    Mamex DC
    Mammomat B
mammography, low-dose
Mammomat B mammography
mandible, mandibular
mandibular notch
maneuver
    flexion
    Valsalva
Mani catheter
Mann-Bollman fistula
manual computed method
manubrium
march foot (fracture)
margin
    colon
    cortical
    disk
    scapular
    stomach
marginal artery of Drummond
marginal osteophyte formation
marginal placenta
marginal serration
marginal spur
marginal ulcer
marginal ulceration

Marie disease
Marie-Bamberger disease
Marie-Tooth disease
Marie-Strümpell disease
marked delay in excretory phase
marked perfusion defect
marker
  nipple
  radiopaque
marker transit study
markings
  bronchovascular
  bronchovesicular
  haustral
  peribronchial
  pulmonary vascular
Marlex mesh
marrow, bone
Martin disease
mass
  discrete
  exophytic
  expansile abdominal
  fluctuant
  hyperdense
  hyperintense
  hypodense
  intra-abdominal
  intraluminal
  low-density
  relativistic
  signal
  soft tissue
  space-occupying
  suspicious
mass effect
masseter muscle
mass lesion
mastectomy, radical
mastication
material, contrast
matrices (pl. of matrix)

matrix, image
matter
  gray
  white
mature pseudocyst of pancreas
maxillary sinus
maxillary spine
maximal radiolucency
Mayer view
Mazer stent
mazoplasia, cystic
McBurney point
mCi (millicurie)
MCP (metacarpophalangeal) joint
MCTC (metrizamide CT cisternogram)
MD-50 contrast medium
MD-60 contrast medium
MD-76 contrast medium
MD-Gastroview contrast medium
meal
  barium
  double contrast barium
  Ewald test
  fatty
  isotope
  motor
  motor test
  opaque
  retention
  small bowel
mean free path
meatus, auditory
mechanism
  deglutition
  propulsive
  swallowing
Meckel diverticulum
Meckel scan
meconium plug
media (pl. of medium)
medial and lateral longitudinal
  reconstruction study

medial compartment
medial condyle of femur
medial condyle of humerus
medial epicondyle fracture
medial femoral condyle
medial lateral ligament of knee
medially
medial patellar facet cartilage
median lethal dose
median raphe
mediastinal node
mediastinal pleura
mediastinal septum
mediastinal thickening
mediastinal wedge
mediastinum
    superior
    widened
mediastinum cerebelli
mediastinum cerebri
mediolateral oblique view
mediolateral stress
mediopatellar
Medi-Tech catheter
medronate scan
medulla oblongata
medullary canal
megacolon
    acquired
    congenital
    idiopathic
    toxic
megaduodenum
megaesophagus of achalasia
megahertz (MHz)
megarectum
meglumine contrast medium
meglumine diatrizoate contrast
    medium
meglumine iodipamide contrast
    medium
meglumine iothalamate contrast
    medium

meglumine iotroxate contrast
    medium
Meigs disease
Meigs syndrome
Meissner plexus
melanoma
melanosarcoma
membrane
    Jackson
    mucous
    synovial
membranes, premature rupture of
membranous pericolitis
Mengert index in pelvimetry
Menghini needle
meningioma
meningocele
meningomyelocele
meniscal injury
meniscus articularis
meniscus lateralis
meniscus medialis
meniscus sign
menses
menstrual date
mental spine
mentoanterior
mentoposterior
mentum
Mercedes-Benz sign
meroacrania
mesenteric
mesenteric node
mesenteric sclerosis
mesenterium commune
mesentery, fatty
mesh, Marlex
mesocuneiform bone
mesocardia
mesocolon
mesoderma
meson

mesosigmoid
mesosternum
mesothelial
metacarpal bone
metacarpophalangeal (MCP) joint
metallic clip
metallic foreign body
metallic long screw fixation device
metaphyseal dysostosis
metaphyseal-epiphyseal angle
metaphysis, metaphyseal
metaplasia
   cartilaginous
   osteocartilaginous
metatases, lymphangitic
metastasis (pl. metastases)
metastatic disease
metatarsal bone
metatarsalgia, Morton
metatarsal head
metatarsal-phalangeal (MTP) joint
metatarsocuneiform joint
metatarsophalangeal (MTP) joint
metatarsus adductocavus deformity
metatarsus adductus deformity
metatarsus atavicus deformity
metatarsus latus deformity
metatarsus primus varus deformity
metatarsus varus deformity
meter, rate
methionine
method
  in vivo
   manual computed
   multiple line scanning
   multiple sensitive point
   multisection
   Pfeiffer-Comberg
   surface coil
methyl methacrylate
metopic suture
metrizamide CT cisternogram

metrizamide myelography
metrizoate sodium contrast medium
metroperitoneal fistula
MHz (megahertz)
microadenoma
microcalcification, clustered
microcardia
microcephaly
microcurie
microdactylia
microfiche
microfocal spot mammogram
midabdominal wall
midaxillary line
midbody
midcolon
middorsal
middle phalanx
middle third of the thoracic
   esophagus
midepigastric area
midepigastrium
midesophageal diverticulum
midfemur
midfoot
midgut volvulus with malrotation
midline shift
midlung field
midpatellar tendon
midpelvis
midpole
midportion
midriff
midshaft fracture
midtarsal
midthigh
Mikulicz angle
miliary tuberculosis
Milkman syndrome (also Looser-
   Milkman)
Miller-Abbott tube
Miller disease
millicurie (mCi)

millijoule
millimeter (mm)
millimeter of mercury (mm Hg)
milliroentgen
Milroy disease
mineralization, bone
mini EKG electrode
minimally displaced fracture
minuscule
minute-sequence study
minute-sequence urogram
misalign
mismatch
misonidazole (radiosensitizer)
mitral area
mitral configuration
mitral orifice
mitral stenosis
mitral valve
Mitsubishi linear accelerator
mm (millimeter)
mm Hg (millimeter of mercury)
mobility
mode
    A-
    B-
    blink
    multiplanar
modified stage exercise
modified radical mastectomy
mole, hydatidiform
Monckeberg calcification
moniliasis
monitor
    cardiac
    Holter
monitoring electrode
monitoring wire
monochromatic radiation
monocular
monodactylism
monomalleolar ankle fracture

Monro bursa
Monteggia dislocation
Monteggia fracture-dislocation
Monteggia fracture of forearm
Monteggia ulna fracture/radial head
    dislocation
Montercaux fracture
Moore fracture
Morand spur
Morel syndrome
Morgagni
    column of
    crypt of
    foramen of
Morgagni hyperostosis
Morgagni-Stewart-Morel syndrome
morphology, morphologic
Morris point
mortise, ankle
mortise joint
Morton metatarsalgia
Morton toe
mosaic pattern of duodenal mucosa
motility, esophageal
motor meal barium GI series
mottled
mottling
movement
    pendulum
    propulsive
    spontaneous fetal
MP articulation
MPD (main pancreatic duct)
MR-cholangiography
MRI (magnetic resonance imaging)
MRS (magnetic resonance spec-
    troscopy)
MSAD (multiple scan average dose)
MSAFP (maternal serum alpha
    fetoprotein)
MTP (metatarsophalangeal) joint
mucocele

mucosa
 antral
 burned out
 cardiac (of stomach)
 cobblestone
 cobblestoning of
 colorectal
 foveolar gastric
 friable
 frothy colonic
 fundic
 intestinal
 normal-appearing
 pyloric
 rectal
 sulciolar gastric
mucosal abnormality
mucosal folds
mucosal island
mucosal pattern
mucosal relief
mucous lake of the stomach
mucous membrane
MUGA (multiple gated acquisition)
 blood pool radionuclide scan
mulberry-type calcification
multangular bone, accessory
multangular ridge fracture
multi-echo axial
multi-echo coronal image
multi-echo image
multi-exponential relaxation
multicentricity
multicystic acoustic neuroma
multigated pulsed Doppler flow
 system
multigravida
multi-interval
multipara
multiparous
multiplanar mode

multiplanar technique
multiple fracture
multiple gated acquisition (MUGA)
 blood pool radionuclide scan
multiple plane imaging
multiple scan average dose (MSAD)
multislice mode
mummy wrapping of children for
 restraint
Münchmeyer disease
mural aneurysm
mural thrombus
Murphy button
muscle
muscular branch
muscularis mucosae
musculature
mushroom-shaped mass
mycetoma
myelin sheath
myelogram
 cervical
 complete
 lumbar
 metrizamide
 positive contrast
 thoracic
myeloma
myenteric plexus of Auerbach
mylohyoid ridge
myocardial infarct imaging
myocardial infarction
myocardial scan
myocarditis
myocardium
myometrium
myositis ossificans
myxedema
myxoma
myxomembranous colitis

# N, n

Nägele obliquity
Nägele pelvis
nail
  cloverleaf
  Jewett
  triflanged
  Zickel
napkin ring annular lesion
napkin ring tumor
naris (pl. nares)
narrowing
  disk space
  joint space
  luminal
  neural foramen
narrowing of artery
  asymmetrical
  symmetrical
nasal sinus
nasal spine
nasion
nasogastric (NG) tube
navel string
navicular
  carpal
  tarsal
naviculocapitate fracture
near anatomic position of joint
neck
  femoral
  pancreatic
  uterine
necrosis
  aseptic
  avascular
  epiphyseal ischemic
  renal cortical

necrosis *(cont.)*
  septic
necrotic tissue
necrotic ulceration
necrotizing enterocolitis
necrotizing vasculitis of bowel
needle
  Amplatz
  Chiba
  coaxial sheath cut-biopsy
  cut-biopsy
  Dos Santos
  fine
  Hawkins
  Jamshidi
  Kopans
  Menghini
  percutaneous
  PermaCut cut-biopsy
  self-aspirating cut-biopsy
  skinny
  spinal
  TruCut biopsy
Nélaton dislocation
Nélaton fold
neocerebellum
neointimal
neonatal
neopallium
neoplasm
  low-grade
  primary
neoplastic fracture
neoplastic stenosis
nephrocalcinosis
nephrolithiasis

nephroptosis
nephrosclerosis, malignant
nephrostogram, post procedure
nephrostomy, Cope
nephrostomy tube
nephrotoxic contrast medium
nerve root
nerve root edema
nerve root sheath
net magnetization factor
neural arch
neural foramen, foramina
neuroangiography
neuroblastoma
neurofibroma
neurofibromatosis
neurogenic arthropathy
neurogenic fracture
neurogenic pulmonary edema
neurogenic tumor
neuroma, multicystic acoustic
Neuropac
NeuroSectOR ultrasound system
neutron
   slow
   thermal
neutron activation analysis
Newton guide wire
NG (nasogastric) tube
niche
   Barclay
   Haudek
nidus
Niemann-Pick disease
nipple marker
NMR (nuclear magnetic resonance)
   scan
NMR spectrum
nodal point
node, nodes
   abdominal
   Aschoff

node *(cont.)*
   axillary
   cervical
   Heberden
   hilar
   hilar lymph
   inguinal
   intramammary
   jugulodigastric
   Keith
   lymph
   mediastinal
   mesenteric
   obturator
   pelvic
   posterior cervical
   regional lymph
   scalene
   Schmorl
   sinoauricular
   Tawara
nodular density
nodular goiter
nodular-like
nodular mass
nodule
   cold
   Gamna
   Gamna-Gandy
   hot
   lingular
   nonfunctioning thyroid
   peripheral
   pulmonary
   siderotic
   solitary pulmonary (SPN)
   thyroid
nonarticular radial head fracture
nondisplaced fracture
nonenhanced CAT scan
nonfunctioning thyroid nodule
nonhomogeneous consolidation

noninfected
noninvasive
nonionic contrast medium
nonlamellated bone
nonobstructive
nonradiopaque foreign body
nonspecific
nontraumatic dislocation
nonunion of fracture fragments
nonunion, torsion wedge
nonvisualization of gallbladder
nonweightbearing
Norland XR26 bone densitometer
normal-appearing mucosa
normal liver parenchyma
notch
   aortic
   cardiac
   clavicular
   coracoid
   costal
   cotyloid
   fibular
   greater sciatic
   interclavicular
   intercondylar
   intercondyloid
   intervertebral
   Kernohan
   lesser sciatic

notch *(cont.)*
   scapular
   sciatic
   sigmoid
   spinoglenoid
   sternal
   trochlear
   ulnar
Novopaque contrast medium
Nuck
   canal of
   diverticulum of
nuclear bone imaging
nuclear magnetic resonance (NMR)
   scan; spectography
nuclear relaxation
nuclear signal
nuclear spin
nuclear spin quantum number
nucleonics
nucleus
   dentate
   Kölliker
nucleus globosus
nucleus pulposus
nuclide
nursemaid's elbow
nutcracker esophagus
nutmeg appearance of liver

# O, o

obelion
oblique diameter of pelvic inlet
oblique fracture
oblique view
obliquity
   Litzmann
   Nägele
   Roederer
   Solayrès
obliterate
obliteration
obscure
obstetric
obstruction
   acute abdominal
   adynamic intestinal
   aortic arch
   biliary
   bowel
   closed-loop intestinal
   colonic
   common bile duct
   common duct
   complete bowel
   esophageal
   extrahepatic
   false colonic
   fecal
   food bolus
   gastric outlet
   hepatic venous outflow
   high small-bowel
   high-grade
   idiopathic
   intestinal
   large-bowel
   low small-bowel
   mechanical biliary

obstruction *(cont.)*
   mechanical duct
   mechanical extrahepatic
   mechanical intestinal
   mechanical small-bowel
   neurogenic intestinal
   paralytic colonic
   partial bowel
   pyloric outlet
   pyloroduodenal
   rectal
   simple mechanical
   small-bowel (SBO)
   strangulated bowel
   strangulation
obstructive component
obstructive emphysema
obturator hernia
obturator nodal chain
obturator node
obtuse marginal (OM) coronary
   artery
occipital bone
occipital fissure
occipital lobe
occipitoanterior
occipitoposterior
occiput
occlude, occlusion
occlusal plane
occlusion, coronary
occult bone metastases
occult fracture
OCG (oral cholecystogram)
octagon board
oculoplethysmography/carotid
   phonoangiography (OPG/CPA)
Oddi sphincter

odontoid bone
odontoid fracture at the base
odontoid fracture at the waist
odontoid process
olecranon
olecranon bursitis
olecranon fossa
olecranon process
oligodactylia
oligodendroglioma
oligohydramnios
Ollier disease
OM (obtuse marginal) coronary
    artery
omentum
    greater
    lesser
omentum minus
Omnipaque, nonionic (iohexol)
omphalic
omphalocele
omphaloma
one-part fracture
onion-shaped dilatation of
    duodenum
onyx
opacification of patent vessel lumen
opacify
opacity
    ground-glass
    linear
opaque media
opaque wire suture
open-break fracture
open dislocation
open fracture
open-mouth odontoid view
open reduction and internal fixation
    (ORIF)
OPG/CPA (oculoplethysmography/
    carotid phonoangiography)
optic globe

optic recess
optimal, optimally
Optiray contrast medium
Optiscope flexible fiberoptic
    angioscope
Orabilex contrast medium
Oragrafin contrast medium
oral cholangiogram
oral cholecystogram (OCG)
orbit, bony
orbital bone
orbitosphenoidal bone
organoaxial
organomegaly
orientation, coronal
ORIF (open reduction and internal
    fixation)
orifice, mitral
Orion balloon catheter
orogastric tube
oropharynx
orthocephalic
orthopnea
orthotonic
os calcis
os coxae
os cuboides secondarium
os epilunatum
os intermetatarseum
os metatarsalia
os naviculare pedis retardatum
os pubis
os sedentarium
os supratalare
os tarsale distale primum
os tarsale distale quartum
os tarsale distale secundum
os tarsale distale tertium
os tarsi fibulare
os tarsi tibiale
os trigonum
os uteri externum

os uteri internum
os vesalianum pedis
Osgood-Schlatter disease
Osler disease
ossa suprasternalia
osseous destructive process
osseous graft
osseous structure
ossicle, Riolan
ossific
ossificans, myositis
ossification
   enchondral
   endochondral
   heterotopic
ossification center, carpal
ossification of muscles
ossifying polymyositis, diffuse
   progressive
osteal
osteitis deformans
osteitis fibrosa cystica
osteitis condensans ilii
osteitis deformans
osteitis fibrosa cystica
osteoarthritis, degenerative
osteoarthropathy, hypertrophic
   pulmonary
osteoarthropathy of fingers, familial
osteoarthrosis
osteoblastic bone regeneration
osteochondral fracture of distal
   radius
osteochondral fragment
osteochondritic separation of
   epiphyses
osteochondritis coxae juvenilis
osteochondritis dissecans
osteochondritis ischiopubica
osteochondroma
osteochondromatosis
osteochondrosis

osteochondrosis deformans juvenilis
osteochondrosis dissecans
osteochondrosis of capital femoral
   epiphysis
osteochondrosis of head of
   metatarsal
osteochondrosis of vertebral
   epiphyses in juveniles
osteoclastic
osteofibromatosis, cystic
osteogenesis, imperfect
osteogenesis imperfecta tarda
osteogenic sarcoma
osteolytic
osteoma
osteomalacia
osteomyelitis
   acute hematogenous
   blastomycotic
   Garre sclerosing
   iatrogenic
   nonsuppurative
   post-traumatic chronic
   sclerosing nonsuppurative
   tuberculous
osteonal bone
osteonecrosis of femoral head
osteopenia
osteoperiostitis of metatarsal
osteopetrosis, autosomal recessive
osteophyte formation, marginal
osteophytes
   bony
   bridging
   fringe of
osteophytic
osteoplastic
osteopoikilosis
osteoporosis, post-traumatic
osteoporotic
osteosarcoma
   parosteal

osteosarcoma *(cont.)*
  periosteal
  telangiectatic
osteosclerosis
ostia
ostium abdominale tubae uterinae
Outerbridge ridge
Outerbridge scale
oval
ovale, foramen
ovarian cyst

overaeration
overexpanded
overhead film; view
overhead oblique view
overlie, overlying
overriding
Overhauser effect
ovoid-shaped
Owen view
oxygen cisternography

# P, p

PA (posteroanterior or posterior-
  anterior)
PA and lateral films; views
Paas disease
pacchionian
pacemaker
pachycephaly
pachydactyly
pad, fat
Paget abscess; disease
pagetoid
Pais fracture
palate, palatal
palate bone
palatine bone
palatopharyngeal fold
palatum durum
palatum fissum
palatum molle
palladium 103 isotope
palpate, palpation
palpebral fissure
Pancoast syndrome
pancreas
  aberrant
  accessory

pancreas *(cont.)*
  annular
  CT scan of
  head of
  heterotopic
  lesser
  neck of
  tail of
  Willis
  Winslow
pancreatic angiography
pancreatic duct
pancreatic duct cannulation, endoscopic retrograde
pancreatic duct disruption
pancreatic pseudocyst
pancreatic scan
pancreaticobiliary common channel
pancreatitis
  calcifying
  centrilobular
  diffuse
  focal
  fulminating
  hemorrhagic necrotizing
  necrotizing

pancreatitis *(cont.)*
   perilobar
   segmentary
pancreatocholangiogram, retrograde
pancreatogram, endoscopic retrograde
panhypopituitarism
panoramic radiography
Panorex x-ray
Pantopaque contrast medium
papilla of duodenum
papilla of Santorini
papilla of Vater
paracentesis
paradoxical hyperconcentration of
   contrast medium
paraesophageal hernia
parahilar
paralytic ileus
paramagnetic relaxation
paramagnetic shift
parameter, sonographic
parametrial spread
paranasal sinus
parapelvic
parapharyngeal space
parasellar
paraspinal
paratracheal stripe
paratrooper fracture
paravertebral
parenchyma
parenchymal collaterals
paries
parietal bone
parietal suture
parieto-occipital
Parona space
parosteal osteosarcoma
parotid gland
parry fracture
pars interarticularis

pars pylorica
partial dislocation
partial saturation and
   spin-echo pulse sequence
particle, beta
partition, gastric
parts, fetal small
passage of blind catheter
patch, Peyer
patchy consolidation
patchy infiltrate
patella
   bipartite
   dislocated
   high-riding
   lower pole of
   minima
   subluxing
   undersurface of
patella alta (high-riding)
patella minima
patellar button
patellar chondromalacia
patellar contour
patellar edge
patellar fat pad
patellar fossa
patellar groove
patellar instability
patellar orthosis pad
patellofemoral joint space
patency, patent
patent ductus arteriosus
patent foramen ovale
patent, patency
patent, widely
pathologic dislocation
pathologic fracture
pathology
pathophysiological change
pattern
   abdominal wall venous

pattern *(cont.)*
  anhaustral colonic gas
  bowel
  bowel gas
  cobblestone
  ductal
  echo
  fold
  gas
  gastric mucosal
  haustral
  homogeneous
  honeycomb
  infiltration
  irregular amputated mucosal
  mosaic duodenal mucosal
  mucosal
  mucosal guideline
  nonspecific gas
  rugal
  signet ring
  small-bowel mucosal
patulous hiatus
paucity
Pawlik trigone
Payr disease
pecten pubis
pectoral
pectus carinatum
pectus excavatum deformity
pedicle
pedunculated polyp
pedunculation
Pel-Ebstein disease
Pellegrini disease
Pellegrini-Stieda calcification
Pellegrini-Stieda disease of knee
pellet, radiopaque
pelvicaliceal (pelvicalyceal)
pelvic bone
pelvic brim
pelvic collateral vessel

pelvic diameter
pelvic floor
pelvic girdle
pelvic inlet
pelvic node
pelvic outlet
pelvic rim fracture
pelvic ring fracture
pelvic sidewall
pelvimetry, Mengert index in
pelvis
  android
  anthropoid
  cordate
  flat
  funnel
  gynecoid
  Kilian
  Nägele
  platypelloid
  portable film of
  renal
  Rokitansky
  small
  spondylolisthetic
pelviureteral junction
penciling of ribs
pendulous breasts
pendulum movement
penetrating ulcer
penoscrotal
Penrose drain
peptic ulcer disease (PUD)
Perchloracap contrast medium
PercuGuide
percutaneous automated diskectomy
percutaneous interventional
  radiology
percutaneous needle
percutaneous retrograde transfemoral technique
percutaneous transhepatic cholangiography (PTC)

percutaneous transluminal angioplasty (PTA)
percutaneous transluminal coronary
angioplasty (PTCA)
percutaneous transluminal renal
angioplasty (PTRA)
perforated diverticulum
perforating aneurysm
perforating fracture
perforating ulcer
perforation
perfuse, perfusion
perfusion abnormality
perfusion defect, marked
perfusion deficit
perfusion lung scan
periampullary diverticulum
periampullary duodenal tumor
periaortic adenopathy
periaortic area
periarticular fracture
peribronchial cuffing
peribronchial infiltrate
peribronchial markings
peribronchiolar
pericallosal artery
pericardial cyst
pericardial effusion
pericardial fat pad
pericardial fluid
pericarditis
pericecal abscess
pericholecystic edema
pericolitis, membranous
periductal calcification
perihilar
perihilar adenopathy
perihilar fibrosis
perihilar infiltrate
perihilar markings
perilunate carpal dislocation
periosteal bone

periosteal sarcoma
periosteal stripping
periosteal thickening
periosteoarthritis of foot
periostitis
peripancreatic area
peripelvic
peripheral fracture
peripheral lung disease
peripheral nodule
periphery
periportal area
perirectal abscess
perirectal spread
perirenal space
perirenal septum
perisigmoid colon
perisinusoidal space
perispondylitis
peristalsis
    absent
    accelerated
    decreased
    increased
    reversed
    visible
peristaltic contraction
peristaltic rush
peristaltic wave
peritendinitis calcarea
peritoneal mouse
peritoneum, peritoneal
peritoneum viscerale
peritonitis
periventricular
perivertebral adenopathy
perivesical
PermaCut cut-biopsy needle
pernicious
peroneal artery
persistence, persistent
pertechnetate

pertrochanteric fracture
perusal
pes abductus
pes adductus
pes arcuatus
pes calcaneus
pes cavus
pes contortus
pes equinovalgus
pes equinovarus
pes excavatus
pes malleus valgus
pes planovalgus
pes planus
pes pronatus
pes supinatus
pes valgus
pes varus
pessary
PET (positron emission tomography) scan
Petit disease
petroclinoid ligament
petrosal bone
petrous bone
petrous portion
petrous pyramid
petrous ridge
Peyer patch
Pfeiffer-Comberg method
phalangeal bones of foot; hand
phalanx (pl. phalanges)
    distal
    middle
    proximal
phantom
    Alderson average-man random
    tissue-equivalent
pharyngoesophageal diverticulum
pharynx, pharyngeal
phase
    wash-in
    washout

phased array study, symmetrical
phase image
phentetiothalein contrast medium
Philips Gyroscan T5
Philips DVI 1 system
Philips tomoscan 350 CT scanner
phlebolith
phlegmon, phlegmonous
photon deficiency
photon-deficient lesion
photon-deficient mass
photopenic area on film or scan
phrenic
phrenoesophageal
phrygian cap
phrygian cap deformity
phthinoid chest
phthisis
physeal plate fracture
physiologic flow
phytobezoar
pia arachnoid
pia mater
Pick bundle
picture element (pixel)
Piedmont fracture
pigeon breast deformity
piggybacking
pillion fracture
pillow fracture
pilonidal cyst
pilonidal sinus
pin
    metallic
    partially threaded
pineal body
pineal gland, calcified
ping-pong fracture
pinhole collimator
PIP (proximal interphalangeal) joint
PIPIDA (P-isopropylacetanilide-
    iminodiacetic acid) scan

Pirie bone
piriform sinus
piriformis muscle
Pirogoff amputation
pisiform bone
pisotriquetral joint
pitchblende
pituitary fossa
pituitary gland
pituitary stalk
pixel (picture element)
placenta, marginal
placenta previa marginalis
placentography
plafond
plain film
planar spin imaging
Planck constant
plane
  axial
  coronal
  fat
  frontal
  horizontal
  imaging
  occlusal
  sagittal
  transverse
  vertical
planography
plantar calcaneal spur
plantar spur
planum popliteum
planum sternale
plaque
  arteriosclerotic
  calcified
  concentric
  eccentric
plaquelike linear defect
plaquing
plate
  compression

plate (cont.)
  cribriform
  end
  epiphyseal
  flat
  growth
  localization-compression grid
plate-and-screw fixation device
plate and screws
plateau fracture
plateau, tibial
platelike atelectasis
platybasia
platycephaly
platypellic pelvis
platypelloid pelvis
platypodia
platyspondyly
pleating of small bowel
plethysmography, impedance (IPG)
pleura
  mediastinal
  visceral
pleural cavity
pleural effusion
pleural fluid
pleural reaction
pleural space
pleural thickening
plexus
  Auerbach
  celiac
  choroid
  Exner
  Meissner
plica (pl. plicae)
Plummer-Vinson syndrome
pneumatic bone
pneumatocele
pneumatosis intestinalis cystica
pneumoconiosis
Pneumocystis carinii

pneumocystography
pneumocystotomography
pneumogastrography
pneumogram, -graphy
  cerebral
  retroperitoneal
pneumogynogram
pneumohemothorax
pneumolith
pneumomediastinography
pneumomediastinum
pneumomyelography
pneumonectomy
pneumonia
  aspiration
  asthmatic
  bacterial
  bronchial
  chronic
  cytomegaloviral
  diffuse
  Friedländer
  granulomatous
  hypostatic
  interstitial
  lingular
  lobar
  mycoplasmal
  pneumococcal
  radiation
  resolving
  respiratory syncytial viral
  unresolved
  viral
pneumonic infiltrate
pneumonitis, radiation
pneumopericardium
pneumoperitoneum
pneumopreperitoneum
pneumopyelography
pneumoradiography
pneumoroentgenogram

pneumothorax, spontaneous
pneumoventriculography
point
  Addison
  Cannon
  Cannon-Boehm
  Clado
  Cope
  Hartmann
  Lanz
  Mackenzie
  McBurney
  nodal
  Morris
point scanning
pole
  inferior
  lower
  middle
  superior
  upper
pole of kidney
pollex pedis
polyarteritis nodosa
polydactylism
polymelia
polyostotic fibrous dysplasia
polyp
  adenomatous
  benign adenomatous
  broad-based
  colonic
  colorectal
  duodenal
  fibrovascular
  hamartomatous gastric
  inflammatory fibroid
  juvenile
  lymphoid
  malignant
  metaplastic
  neoplastic

polyp *(cont.)*
   pedunculated
   Peutz-Jeghers
   postinflammatory
   rectal
   retention
   sessile
   stalk of
   tubular
   tubulovillous
   villous
polypoid filling defect
polypoid lesion
polyposis intestinalis
polyp stalk
pond fracture
pons
pontine angle
pool, vascular blood
poor visualization
popliteal aneurysm
popliteal artery; vein
popliteal space
porcelain gallbladder
porencephaly
porencephalic cyst
porosis
portable chest x-ray
portable film
portable pelvis x-ray
portable vascular bed
porus acusticus externus osseus
position
   anatomic
   anterior oblique
   Bertel
   decubitus
   dorsal
   dorsal lithotomy
   dorsal recumbent
   erect
   Fowler

polyp *(cont.)*
   frogleg
   Gaynor-Hart
   LAO (left anterior oblique)
   lateral
   lateral decubitus
   left lateral decubitus
   lordotic
   LPO (left posterior oblique)
   Mayer
   near anatomic
   normal anatomic
   prone
   RAO (right anterior oblique)
   recumbent
   reverse Trendelenburg
   RPO (right posterior oblique)
   scissor leg
   semi-Fowler
   Sims
   spinal fusion
   Statue of Liberty (in spica cast)
   steep Trendelenburg
   supine
   swimmer's
   Trendelenburg
   Walcher
   wedge
position of joint, near anatomic
positron emission tomography
   (PET)
postangioplasty aortogram
postcubital
postdilatation
postdilatation arteriogram
posterior-anterior (PA)
posterior cervical node
posterior cervical triangle
posterior elements
posterior facet joint
posterior-lateral
posterior lip

posterior-medial
posterior segment
posterior spur
posterior sulcus
posterior tibial artery
posteroanterior (PA)
posterolateral
posterolateral aspect
posteromedial
postevacuation view
postlymphangiography
postoperative pancreatitis
postradiation fibrosis
postprocedure nephrostogram
postsphenoidal bone
poststenotic dilatation
postsurgical
post-transplant acute renal failure
   (ARF)
post-traumatic arthritis
post-traumatic osteomyelitis of skull
post-traumatic osteoporosis
postulnar bone
postvoid(ing) film
postvoid residual (PVR)
potassium perchlorate contrast
   medium
Pott disease
Pott fracture
potter's asthma
pouch
   blind
   Kock
   Rathke
   Zenker
Poupart ligament
precession
precessional frequency
precipitate evacuation
predominance, predominant
prefrontal bone of von Bardeleben

pregnancy
   abdominal
   ectopic
   extrauterine
   gemellary
   heterotopic
   intrauterine
   tubal
Preiser disease
preliminary film; view
premature rupture of membranes
prep (preparation), bowel
prepatellar bursa
preponderance
prepontine cistern
prepped
prepyloric atresia
prepyloric fold
prerenal
presbyarthritis
presbyesophagus
presentation of fetus
   breech
   brow
   cephalic
   compound
   face
   footling
   frank breech
   parietal
   shoulder
   transverse
   vertex
presenting part
presphenoidal bone
pressure fracture
pressure gradient
pressure study
prevertebral adenopathy
primary complex
primary neoplasm
primitive dislocation

principle, uncertainty
Priodax contrast medium
probe
  biplane sector
  ultrasound
procedure, Ripstein
process, processes
  alveolar consolidative
  articular
  bony
  coracoid
  coronoid
  costal
  glenoid
  inflammatory
  knobby
  lumbar transverse
  neoplastic
  odontoid
  olecranon
  osseous destructive
  pterygoid
  sacral
  spinous
  styloid
  transverse
  trochlear
  vermiform
  vertebral
  xiphoid
  zygomatic
processus costarius vertebrae
processus lateralis tali
processus lateralis tuberis calcanei
processus medialis tuberis calcanei
processus xiphoideus
proctogram, video
profunda femoris
prognathic dilatation
project, projected
projection (see *view)*
prolactinoma

prolapse
prominence, prominent
promontory, sacral
pronation
prone position
prone view
proportional counter
propulsive mechanism
propyliodone contrast medium
prosthesis, prostheses
  acetabular
  femoral
  total hip replacement
  total knee replacement
protocol, urokinase
proton density image
protrude
protrusion, spicular
proximal
proximal anterior tibial artery
proximal arterial tree
proximal interphalangeal (PIP) joint
Pruitt-Inahara carotid shunt
psammoma, Virchow
pseudocoarctation of aorta
pseudocoxalgia
pseudocyst, mature pancreatic
pseudodextrocardia
pseudodislocation
pseudoepiphysis
pseudoextrophy
pseudofracture
pseudogout
pseudohaustration
pseudoluxation
pseudo-obstruction, idiopathic
  intestinal
pseudopolyp
pseudopregnancy
pseudotumor
psoas muscle
psoas shadow

PTA (percutaneous transluminal angioplasty)
PTC (percutaneous transhepatic cholangiography)
PTCA (percutaneous transluminal coronary angioplasty)
pterion
pterygoideus hamulus
pterygoid bone
ptosis, ptotic
PTRA (percutaneous transluminal renal angioplasty)
pubic bone
pubic ramus (pl. rami)
　inferior
　superior
pubic symphysis
pubic tubercle
pubococcygeal line
PUD (peptic ulcer disease)
pulled elbow
pulmonary angiogram
pulmonary artery
pulmonary contusion
pulmonary edema
pulmonary embolism; embolus
pulmonary emphysema
pulmonary fibrosis
pulmonary infiltrate
pulmonary nodule
pulmonary perfusion and ventilation
pulmonary stenosis
pulmonary tuberculosis
pulmonary vascular congestion
pulmonary vascular markings
pulmonary vascular redistribution
pulmonary vein
pulposus, nucleus

pulsate
pulsed gradient
pulse amplifier
pulse indicator, xylol
pulse length
pulse radiofrequency
pulse sequence
pulse width
pulsing current
punctum coxale
punctum ischiadicum
puncture, dural
purpura, Henoch
PVR (postvoiding residual)
pyelectasis
pyelocaliceal
pyelocaliectasis
pyelocalyceal
pyelofluoroscopy
pyelogram, intravenous (IVP)
pyelography, antegrade
pyelonephritis
pyknodysostosis
pyloric channel, eccentric
pyloric hypertrophy
pyloric insufficiency
pyloric stenosis
pyloric string sign
pyloric ulcer
pyloric valve
pylorospasm, persistent
pylorus
PYP (pyrophosphate) technetium scan
pyramid, petrous
pyramidal bone
pyramidal fracture (of maxilla)
pyrophosphate

# Q, q

QCT (quantitative computed
    tomography)
Quad-Lumen radiopaque drain
quadrant
quadrature detector
quadrigeminal
quality factor
quantitative computed tomography
    (QCT)

quantitative exercise thallium 201
    variables
quantum number
quantum theory
quench, quenching
Quervain (de Quervain) disease
Quervain fracture

# R, r

R (roentgen)
R meter
rad (radiation absorbed dose)
radiability
radial bone
radial fossa
radial head
radial tuberosity
radiation
    Cerenkov
    monochromatic
radiation cystitis
radiation pneumonitis
radical mastectomy
radical prostatectomy
radicle, biliary
radiculopathy
Radiofocus Glidewire for angi-
    ography
radioactive bolus
radioactive iodinated serum
    albumin (RISA) study

radioactive marker
radioactive tracer
radiocarpal angle
radiochemistry
radiofrequency (RF) coil; pulse
radiograph
radiographic changes
radiography
radiohumeral bursitis
radioimmunodetection (RAID)
radioisotope (isotope)
    Ga 67 (gallium citrate)
    Gd-DTPA
    $^{123}$I (sodium iodide) (iodine 123)
    $^{131}$I (sodium iodide) (iodine 133)
    Indium 111
    $^{99m}$technetium sodium
        pertechnetate
    technetium 99m (Tc 99m)
    technetium 99m albumin colloid
    technetium 99m albumin
    microspheres

radioisotope *(cont.)*
  technetium 99m DISIDA
  technetium 99m DMSA
  technetium 99m DTPA
  technetium 99m DTPA aerosol
  technetium 99m GHP
  technetium 99m HDP
  technetium 99m HIDA
  technetium 99m labeled A.C.
  technetium 99m labeled stannous
    methylene diphosphonate
  technetium 99m lidofenin
  technetium 99m MAA
  technetium 99m MDP
  technetium 99m medronate
  technetium 99m pentetic acid
  technetium 99m PIPIDA
  technetium 99m polyphosphate
  technetium 99m PYP (pyro-
    phosphate)
  technetium 99m sodium pertech-
    netate
  technetium 99m sulfur colloid
  thallium 201 (Tl 201)
  xenon 133 (Xe 133)
radioisotope labeling
radiology
  interventional
  percutaneous interventional
radiolucency
radiolucent
radionuclide angiocardiogram
radionuclide labeling
radionuclide liver scan
radionuclide milk scan
radionuclide spleen scan
radiopacity
radiopaque calculus
radiopaque bone cement, Surgical
  Simplex P
radiopaque contrast medium
radiopaque marker

radiopaque pellet
radiopaque suture
radiosensitizer
radiotherapy, upper mantle
radius, radial
radix pulmonis
RAID (radioimmunodetection)
ramus (pl. rami)
  inferior
  pubic
  superior
Ranke angle
RAO (right anterior oblique)
  position
raphe, median
rapid sequential CT scan
rarefied area
rate meter
Rathke pouch
ratio
  cardiothoracic (CT)
  contrast-to-noise (C/N)
  magnetogyric
  signal-to-noise (S/N)
Rau, apophysis of
ray, grenz
rCBF (regional cerebral blood flow)
rCBV (regional cerebral blood
  volume)
rd (rutherford) unit
RDG (retrograde duodenogastroscopy)
reabsorption, bony
reaction
  endoergic
  exoergic
  hilar
  pleural
reading, wet x-ray
re-bypass
real-time assessment
real-time Color Flow Doppler

real-time equipment
real-time image
real-time sonogram
real-time ultrasound
real-time ultrasonography
receiver coil
recess
    intersigmoid
    optic
    sacciform
Recklinghausen disease of bone
reconstituted
reconstituted via collaterals
reconstitution
recovery time
recovery, saturation
rectal fold
rectilinear bone scan
rectilinear thyroid scan
rectosigmoid
rectovaginal septum
rectum, rectal
rectus abdominis muscle
recumbent position; view
recur, recurred, recurrence
recurvatum deformity
Redifurl TaperSeal IAB catheter
redistribution, pulmonary vascular
redistribution study
reflux
    duodenogastric
    duodenopancreatic
    gastric
    gastroesophageal (GER)
    hepatojugular
    vesicoureteral
reflux bile gastritis
reflux esophagitis
reflux regurgitation
regional cerebral blood flow (rCBF)
    study
regional cerebral blood volume
    (rCBV)

regional ileitis
regional lymph nodes
regional pulmonary perfusion
regress, regression
regurgitation
Rehfuss test
Rehfuss tube
Reid baseline
relativistic mass
relaxation
    ferromagnetic
    nuclear
    paramagnetic
    spin-lattice
    spin-spin
relaxation rate
relaxation time
relief pattern
relief, mucosal
remodeling of bone
renal agenesis
renal angiogram
renal artery
renal artery occlusion
renal artery stenosis
renal calculus
renal cortical necrosis
renal lithiasis (renolithiasis)
renal parenchymal disease
renal pelvis
renal shadow
renal sinus echo
renal vein
Renografin contrast medium
renography, DTPA
renolithiasis (renal lithiasis)
Reno-M-Dip contrast medium
Reno-M-60 contrast medium
Reno-M-30 contrast medium
Renovist II contrast medium
Renovue-Dip contrast medium
repeated FID (free induction decay)
repetition time (TR)

rephasing gradient
replacement bone
replacement, fatty
reprepped
resecting fracture
resection
residual, residuum
   fibrocalcific
   fibrocystic
   fibrotic
   gastric
   postvoid
   postvoiding (PVR)
residual contrast material
residual interstitial changes
residue, fecal
resolution
   contrast
   interval
   spatial
resolving time
resorption, bony
resorption phase of healing
respiratory atrium
respiratory compensation
result
   false-negative
   false-positive
resurrection bone
retained secretions
rete ridge
reticular infiltrate
reticuloendothelial
reticulum
retraction, nipple
retroareolar dysplasia
retroappendiceal fossa
retrocalcaneal spur
retrocardiac
retrocecal appendix
retroflexion
retrograde aortogram
retrograde atherectomy

retrograde atrial activation mapping
retrograde filling
retrograde flow
retrograde duodenogastroscopy
   (RDG)
retrograde transfemoral aortography
retrograde urethrogram
retroperitoneal fibrosis
retroperitoneal malignancy
retroperitoneal space
retropulsion of bone fragment into
   spinal canal
retrosternal thyroid
Retzius
   line of
   space of
reverse Barton fracture
reverse Colles fracture
reversed Mercedes-Benz sign
reversed peristalsis
reversible airways disease
Reye syndrome
RF (radiofrequency) coil
rhabdomyosarcoma
rhebosis
rheumatic valvular disease
rheumatoid arthritis
rheumatoid spondylitis
rhomboid ligament
rhythmic segmentation
rib (pl. ribs)
   bicipital
   cervical
   false
   floating
   penciling of
   rudimentary
   slipping
   sternal
   Stiller
   true
   vertebrocostal
   vertebrosternal

Richter hernia
rider's bone
ridge
    mylohyoid
    Outerbridge
    petrous
Riedel lobe
right anterior oblique (RAO)
    position
Rieux hernia
right lower lobe (RLL) of lung
right middle lobe (RML) of lung
right posterior oblique (RPO)
    position
right-to-left shift
right upper lobe (RUL) of lung
right ventricular hypertrophy (RVH)
Rigiflex balloon dilator
rim
    high-density
    low-density
ring, Cannon
Ring catheter
ring fracture
Ring-McLean catheter
ring, Schatzki
Riolan, arch of
Riolan bone
Riolan ossicle
RISA (radioactive iodinated serum
    albumin) study
RLL (right lower lobe) of lung
RML (right middle lobe) of lung
RNA (radionuclide angiogram),
    gated
RNV (radionuclide ventriculogram)
rod, TLD (thermoluminescent
    dosimeter)
Roederer obliquity
roentgen (R)
roentgenkymography
roentgenogram, -graphy

roentgenologist
ROI (region of interest)
Rokitansky-Ashoff sinus
Rokitansky diverticulum
Rokitansky pelvis
Rolando, fissure of
Rolando fracture
rollbewegung rush (German "rolling
    movement")
roof, acetabular
root
    aortic
    nerve
root of the lung
ropy
Rosch catheter
rostrum of the corpus callosum
rostrum sphenoidale
rotary scoliosis
rotary thoracolumbar scoliosis
rotating frame imaging
rotating frame of reference
rotator cuff tear
rotoscoliosis
routine study; view
RPO (right posterior oblique)
    position
Rubin test
rudiment
rudimentary bone
rudimentary rib
rudimentary sinus
ruga, rugae
rugae gastricae
rugal fold
rugal pattern
RUL (right upper lobe) of lung
rule out
runoff
    aortofemoral
    arterial
    peripheral

runoff vessel
ruptured disk
rush
    peristaltic
    rolbewegung

rutherford (rd) unit
Ruysch disease
RVH (right ventricular hypertrophy)

# S, s

S1–S5 (five sacral vertebrae)
saber shin
sac
    amniotic
    dural
    thecal
sacciform recess
saccule
sacculus ventricularis
sacral promontory
sacralization
sacrococcygeal joint
sacroiliac articulation
sacroiliac disease
sacroiliac (SI) joint
sacroiliac subluxation
sacropubic diameter
sacrosciatic foramen
sacrosciatic notch
sacrouterine
sacrovertebral angle
sacrum
sagittal groove
sagittal orientation
sagittal plane
sagittal section
sagittal sinus
sagittal suture
salpingectomy
salpingogram, -graphy
salpinx (pl. salpinges)

Salpix contrast medium
Salter fracture
Salter-Harris type II fracture
SAM (scanning acoustic micro-
    scope)
SAM (systolic anterior motion)
Santorini duct
Santorini, papilla of
sarcoid of Boeck
sarcoma
    osteogenic
    periosteal
saturation recovery
saturation recovery technique
saturation transfer
sawtooth appearance
saw-toothed appearance
SBO (small-bowel obstruction)
SBFT (small-bowel follow-through)
SBO (spina bifida occulta)
scale
    gray
    false color
scalene node
scalloping of vertebrae
scan, scanning
    axial
    B-
    bile duct
    B-mode
    bone

scan *(cont.)*
  brain
  cardiac
  CAT (computerized axial tomography)
  cine CT (computerized tomography)
  color Doppler
  Compuscan Hittman computerized
  computed transmission tomography
  contiguous
  contrast material, enhanced
  CT (computerized tomography)
  CTAT (computerized transverse axial tomography)
  dipyridamole thallium 201
  DISIDA
  Doppler
  duplex
  duplex Doppler (duplex DS)
  flow
  gallbladder
  gallium
  gated equilibrium blood pool
  indium 111 labeled leukocyte
  isotope
  isotope labeled fibrinogen leg
  liver
  liver-spleen
  lung
  medronate
  MRI (magnetic resonance imaging)
  MUGA (multiple gated acquisition) blood pool radionuclide
  myocardial
  NMR (nuclear magnetic resonance)
  oblique
  pancreatic

scan *(cont.)*
  perfusion lung
  PET (positron emission tomography)
  PIPIDA
  point
  radionuclide milk
  rectilinear bone
  redistributed thallium
  resting MUGA
  rest thallium 201
  R-to-R
  SPECT thallium
  stacked
  STIR (short T1 inversion recovery)
  stress thallium
  technetium 99m pyrophosphate myocardial
  thallium
  thyroid
  total body
  triple phase bone
  TSPP rectilinear bone
  ultrafast CT
  unenhanced
  venous
  ventilation
  ventilation-perfusion (VQ)
scanhead
scanner
  Aloka ultrasound linear
  Aloka ultrasound sector
  ATL Mark 600 real-time sector
  ATL real-time NeuroSectOR
  Compuscan Hittman computerized electrocardioscanner
  EMI CT
  GE 8800 CT
  GE 9800 high-resolution CT
  high field strength
  Imatron C-100 ultrafast CT

scanner *(cont.)*
    Philips tomoscan 350 CT
    Siemens Somaform 512 CT
    Siemens Somatom DR2 whole-
      body; also DR3
    Toshiba TCT-80 CT
    UM 4 real-time sector
scan time
scan with contrast enhancement
scan without contrast enhancement
scaphoid bone
scaphoiditis, Köhler tarsal
scapholunate dissociation
scapholunate widening
scapular bone
scapular notch
scarred duodenum
scarring
    basilar pleural
    parenchymal
    pleural
scatoma (stercoroma)
scattering, coherent
Schanz disease
Schatzki ring
Scheuermann disease
Schlatter disease
Schlatter-Osgood disease
Schmorl disease
Schmorl node
Schüller disease
Schüller view
Schwartz introducer
scirrhous carcinoma
sciatic notch
scintigraphic study
scintigraphy
    $^{131}$I MIBG
    isotope
scintillation camera
scintillation detector

scintiphoto(graph)
scintiscan
scintiscanning, adrenal
sclerosing nonsuppurative osteo-
    myelitis
sclerosis
    subchondral
    mesenteric
sclerotic
scoliosis
    dextroscoliosis
    levoscoliosis
    lumbar
    rotary
    S-shaped
    thoracic
    thoracolumbar
scout film; view
scout negative film
screen-film mammogram
screw
    cancellous
    metallic
    transfixing
    Venable
screw and plate
scrobiculus cordis
scrotal hernia
scybalum (pl. scybala)
SE (spin-echo) image
seat belt injury
secondary fracture
second portion of the duodenum
section
    axial
    cesarean
    coronal
    sagittal
    transverse
sector probe, biplane
sector scanning

segment
  posterior
  superior
segmental atelectasis
segmental bone loss
segmental defect
segmental fracture
segmentation
  Cannon
  rhythmic
Segond fracture
Seikosha video printer for scans
Seldinger catheter
Seldinger technique
selective excitation
selective injection
selective irradiation
selective visceral arteriography
self-aspirating cut-biopsy needle
sella turcica
semicircular canal
semilunar bone
semilunar bony formation
semilunar valve
senile ankylosing hyperostosis
  of spine
senile coxitis
senile subcapital fracture
Senographe 500 T mammography
sensitive plane
sensitive plane projection
  reconstruction imaging
sensitive point scanning
sensitize, sensitization
sensitized blood
sensitometer
sentinel loop
separation
septic necrosis
septum
  interatrial
  interlobar

septum (cont.)
  interventricular
  mediastinal
  perirenal
  rectovaginal
septum auricularum
septum pellucidum
sequence
  Carr-Purcell
  Carr-Purcell-Meiboom-Gill
  partial saturation
  pulsed
  spin-echo pulse
  voiding
sequence time
sequential plane imaging
sequential point imaging
sequestrum, sequestra
series
  acute abdominal
  dynamic
  sinus
  small-bowel
  upper GI (gastrointestinal)
SER-IV (supination, external
  rotation-type IV) fracture
serration, marginal
sesamoid bone
sessile tumor
setting, wide window
Sever disease
SFA (superficial femoral artery)
S-FDF (ferrioxamine)
shadow, shadowing
  acoustic
  breast
  iliopsoas muscle
  renal
  snowstorm
shaft
  bone
  French

shaped
  barrel-
  dumbbell-
  ovoid-
  S-
  spheroid-
shear fracture
sheath
  Henle
  myelin
  nerve root
sheetlike
Shepherd fracture
shield, Faraday
shift
  chemical
  Doppler frequency
  left-to-right
  midline
  paramagnetic
  right-to-left
shim coil
shimming
shin bone
short-arm Grollman catheter
short bone
short head
short T1 inversion recovery (STIR)
short TR/TE (T1 weighted image)
shortening of phalanges
shunt
  Denver hydrocephalus
  Denver peritoneal venous
sialography CT
sickle cell anemia
sickle-shaped fold
sideropenic dysphagia
siderotic nodules in the spleen
siderotic splenomegaly
sideswipe elbow fracture
sidewinder catheter
Siemens Somaform 512 CT scanner

Siemens Somatom DR2 whole-body
  scanner (also DR3)
sigma elongatum
sigma in alto fixatum
sigmoid cavity
sigmoid colon
sigmoid curve
sigmoid notch
sigmoid valve
sign
  ace of spades (on angiogram)
  Allis
  Babinski
  barber pole
  bowler hat
  chain of lakes
  double-bubble duodenal
  inverted V
  meniscus
  Mercedes-Benz
  piston
  Spalding
  steeple
  Stierlin
  string of pearls
  Terry-Thomas
  tethered bowel
  Thurston Holland
  windshield wiper
signal acquisitions
signal, Doppler flow
signal intensity
signal mass
signal-to-noise ratio (S/N)
signet ring pattern
SI (sacroiliac) joint
silent gallstone
silhouette
  cardiac
  cardiovascular
silicosis
silver-fork deformity

silver-fork fracture
Sims position
Simmons 1 catheter
Simmons 2 catheter
Simmons 3 catheter
simple dislocation
simple fracture, complex
simultaneous volume imaging
sinciput
single contrast study
single peak
single photon absorptiometry (SPA)
single photon emission computed
    tomography (SPECT)
sinoatrial node
sinoauricular node
Sinografin contrast medium
sinus
    accessory
    draining
    ethmoid
    frontal
    maxillary
    nasal
    paranasal
    pilonidal
    piriform
    renal
    Rokitansky-Aschoff
    rudimentary
    sagittal
    sphenoid
    thickened
sinus cavernosus
sinusitis
sinus of Valsalva
sinus series
sinus tract
site
site of arterial puncture
situs inversus
situs perversus

situs solitus
situs transversus
size and caliber
size and configuration
skeletal disruption
skeletal hypoplasia
skeletal survey, isotopic
skeleton, bony
skier's fracture
Skillern fracture
skin depth
skinny needle
skin thickening
Skiodan contrast medium
skull base
skull, cloverleaf
skull films
skyline view of patella
slice
    tissue
    tomographic
slice thickness
sliding-type hiatal hernia
slow neutron
small-bowel contents
small-bowel follow-through (SBFT)
small-bowel series
small-bowel transit time
smear fragment
Smith dislocation
Smith fracture
S/N (signal-to-noise) ratio
snowstorm shadow
snuffbox, anatomic
sodium diatrizoate contrast medium
sodium iodide contrast medium
sodium iodohippurate contrast
    medium
sodium iodomethamate contrast
    medium
sodium iothalamate contrast
    medium

sodium ipodate contrast medium
sodium methiodal contrast medium
sodium pertechnetate
sodium thorium tartrate contrast
    medium
sodium tyropanoate contrast
    medium
softening and swelling of cartilage
soft palate
soft tissue abnormality
soft tissue calcification
soft tissue density
soft tissue interposition
soft tissue, stippled
soft tissue swelling
Solayrès obliquity
solid bone
solid lesion, echogenic
solitary pulmonary nodule (SPN)
Somatom DR CT scanner
Sones technique of selective
    coronary arteriography
sonogram
    fatty meal (FMS)
    real-time
sonographic parameter
sonography
    Acuson computed
    Acuson transvaginal
    duplex pulsed-Doppler
sonolucent cystic lesion or mass
sonolucent fluid-filled area
SPA (single photon absorptiometry)
space
    disk
    foraminal
    intervertebral disk
    joint
    Kiernan
    parapharyngeal
    perirenal
    pleural

space *(cont.)*
    popliteal
    subarachnoid
    Zang
space-occupying lesion
space of Retzius
Spalding sign
spare, sparing
spasm, esophageal
spasticity
spatial peak intensity
SPECT (single photon emission
    computed tomography) scan
spectography, nuclear magnetic
    resonance (NMR)
spectrometer
spectroscopy, magnetic resonance
    (MRS)
Spence, tail of
sphenocephaly
sphenoid bone
sphenoid sinus
sphenoparietal suture
sphenoturbinal bone
spheroid-shaped
sphincter ani
sphincter muscle
sphincter of Oddi
spicular protrusion
spicule of bone
spiderweb appearance
spin coupling
spin density, echo
spin echo (SE)
spin-echo image
spin-echo pulse sequence
spin-echo sequence
spin-lattice relaxation
spin-spin relaxation
spin-warp imaging
spina bifida occulta (SBO)
spina iliaca

spina ischiadica
spina meatus
spinal canal
spinal column
spinal cord
spinal fusion
spinal instability
spinal muscular atrophy
spindle, His
spine
    anterior maxillary
    cervical (C)
    Charcot
    coccygeal
    dorsal (D)
    iliac
    ischial
    lumbar (L)
    lumbosacral (LS)
    mandibular
    maxillary
    mental
    nasal
    poker
    posterior-inferior
    sacral (S)
    thoracic (T)
    thoracolumbar
    trochanteric
spinoglenoid notch
spinous process
spiral fracture
spiral oblique fracture
splanchnic
splash, succussion
splaying
spleen
splenic flexure
splenization
splenography
splenomegaly, siderotic
splenulus

splint bone
split-compression fracture
splitting, zero-field
SPN (solitary pulmonary nodule)
spoke bone
spondylitis
    ankylosing
    rheumatoid
spondylitis deformans
spondylolisthesis
    sagittal roll
    slip angle
spondylolisthetic pelvis
spondylolysis
spondylosis
spondylosyndesis
sponge
    Ivalon
    Vistec
spongy bone
spontaneous fracture
spontaneous pneumothorax
spot film; view
SPP (superparamagnetic particle)
    contrast medium
sprain fracture
spread, transfascial
Sprengel deformity
sprinter's fracture
spur
    acromial
    bone
    bony
    calcaneal
    degenerative
    heel
    Morand
    plantar
    plantar calcaneal
    posterior
    retrocalcaneal

spurring
  anterior
  hypertrophic marginal
  inferior
  marginal
S-shaped scoliosis
SSFP (steady state free precession)
stable isotope
stacked scans
stage of exercise, modified
staghorn calculus
staging, Greulich and Pyle skeletal
  maturation
stairstep fracture
stalk, pituitary
standoff
stasis, gallbladder
stasis, static
static image
static in appearance
status post
steady state free precession (SSFP)
steatorrhea
steep Towne projection
steeple sign
stellate fracture
stellate skull fracture
stem, brain
stenosis
  bronchial
  concentric hourglass
  focal
  high-grade
  mitral
  neoplastic
  renal artery
  spinal
stenotic
stent
  antegrade ureteral
  biliary
  Carey-Coons

stent *(cont.)*
  Mazer
  patent
  ureteral
Stenver views
stercoroma
stercoral ulcer
stereoscopic film; view
stereotactic (or stereotaxic) data
stereotaxic guide, BRW CT
stereotaxic procedure
stereotaxy
sterile, sterilely
sternal angle
sternal notch
Sternberg disease
sternoclavicular angle
sternocleidomastoid muscle
Stensen duct
Stewart-Hamilton equation
Stewart-Morel syndrome
Stieda disease
Stierlin sign
stiffening
Still disease
Stiller rib
stippled calcification
stippled soft tissue
STIR (short T1 inversion recovery)
  scan
stomach
  bilocular
  cardiac
  cascade
  cup-and-spill
  distended
  dumping
  greater curvature of
  Holzknecht
  hourglass
  intrathoracic
  leather bottle

stomach *(cont.)*
  lesser curvature of
  riding
  thoracic
  trifid
  waterfall
  water-trap
stone
  gall
  kidney
stopcock
strain fracture
strandy infiltrate
strawberry gallbladder
straw-colored
stress cystogram
stress fracture
stress-type fracture
stricture
string of pearls sign
string sign
stripe
  paratracheal
  vertebral
structure
  bony
  high-density
  KUB
  low-contrast
  low-density
  osseous
  renal collecting
  tubular
  vascular
Strümpell disease
Strümpell-Marie disease
studding, endometriosis
study (see also *view)*
  air contrast
  anisotropic 3-D
  AP (anteroposterior)
  blood flow

study *(cont.)*
  contrast
  Cytomel suppression
  double contrast
  flow
  inhalation
  isotropic 3-D
  limited
  marker transit
  medial and lateral longitudinal
    reconstruction
  outside
  PA (posteroanterior)
  postcontrast
  poststress
  pre-contrast
  pressure
  radiographically normal
  redistribution
  tomographic
  volume
Sturge-Weber disease
styloid process
subapical
subarachnoid space
subareolar
subastragalar dislocation
subcapital fracture
  impacted
  senile
subcarinal
subcarinal adenopathy
subchondral plate
subchondral sclerosis
subclavian artery
subclavian catheter
subclavian steal syndrome
subclavian vein
subclavicular
subcoracoid dislocation of shoulder
subcortical
subcutaneous air

subcutaneous emphysema
subcutaneous fat line
subcutaneous fracture
subcutaneous tissue
subdiaphragmatic
subdural blood
subdural hematoma
subdural hemorrhage
subglenoid dislocation of shoulder
subhepatic
sublux, subluxed
subluxated
subluxation
    forward
    Volkmann
subluxing patella
submaxillary
submental vertex view
suboptimal
subperiosteal abscess of frontal sinus
subperiosteal fracture
subperiosteally
subphrenic
subpubic arch
subsegmental bibasilar atelectasis
subspinous dislocation
substernal goiter
substitution bone
subtalar joint
subtraction films
subtraction technique
subtrochanteric fracture
succenturiate
Sudeck atrophy
sulci, cortical
sulcus (pl. sulci)
    angularis
    basilar
    blunted posterior
    costal
    Harrison
sulfur colloid labeled with $^{99m}$Tc

superficial femoral artery (SFA)
superimpose, superimposition
superior mediastinum
superior pubic ramus (pl. rami)
superior pulmonary artery
superior segment
superior vena cava
supernumerary bone
superolaterally
superomedial portal
supination
supine full view
supine position; view
supplementary
suppression, Cytomel
suppurative
supracondylar femoral fracture
supracondylar fracture
supracondylar humerus fracture
supraepicondylar
supraepitrochlear
suprainterparietal bone
supraoccipital bone
supraorbital
suprapatellar bursa
suprapatellar bursal region
suprapharyngeal bone
suprapubic area
suprarenal extension of aneurysm
suprarenal gland
suprasellar lesion
suprasellar mass
supraspinatus
suprasternal bone
supratrochlear
supravaterian duodenum
supraventricular
surface coils
surgical clips
surgical neck of humerus
Surgical Simplex P radiopaque bone
    cement

survey, metastatic bone
suspension, barium
sutural bone
sutural diastasis
suture, sutures
   biparietal
   coronal
   cranial
   dentate
   frontal
   lambdoid
   metopic
   opaque wire
   overlapping
   parietal
   radiopaque
   sagittal
   sphenoparietal
   surgical
   wire
swallow, barium
swallowing function
swallowing mechanism
Swan-Ganz catheter
Swediaur disease
sweep, duodenal
swelling, soft tissue
swimmer's view
sylvian fissure
Sylvius, aqueduct of
Syme amputation
symmetrical narrowing of artery
symmetrical phased array
symmetry
symphysis, pubic
symphysis pubis
syndactyly
syndrome
   afferent loop
   Ayerza
   anterior compartment
   Beau

syndrome *(cont.)*
   blue toe
   Boerhaave
   carpal tunnel
   Chilaiditi
   compartment
   cubital tunnel
   Dandy-Walker
   dumping
   empty sella
   Goodpasture
   Holt-Oram
   irritable bowel
   Loeffler
   Looser-Milkman
   Lutembacher
   Meig
   Milkman
   Morel
   Morgagni-Stewart-Morel
   Pancoast
   patellar malalignment
   Plummer-Vinson
   temporomandibular joint (TMJ)
   Stewart-Morel
   subclavian steal
synostosis
system
   biliary
   caliceal
   collecting
   external jugular
   hepatic ductal
   internal carotid
   intrahepatic
   renal collecting
   reticuloendothelial
   upper collecting
   ventricular
synovial fluid; membrane
synovitis, chronic
systolic anterior motion (SAM)

# T, t

T (tesla)
T (thoracic) spine
T1–T12 (12 thoracic vertebrae)
T condylar fracture
T fracture
T-shaped fracture
T-tube cholangiogram
T1 or $T_1$ (longitudinal or spin-lattice relaxation time constant)
T1 or $T_1$ weighted coronal image
T1 or $T_1$ weighted image (short TR/TE)
T1 or $T_1$ weighted sagittal image
T2 or $T_2$ (spin-spin or transverse relaxation time)
T2 or $T_2$ (transverse or spin-spin relaxation time constant)
T2 or $T_2$ time constant
T2 or $T_2$ weighted image (long TR/TE)
T2 or $T_2$ weighted spin-echo image
$T_4$ RIA (thyroxine radioisotope assay)
3DFT (3-dimensional Fourier transform) magnetic resonance angiography
table swivel
taenia choroidea
taenia coli
taenia omentalis
taenia terminalis
taeniae pylori
tag
tagged atom
tail of breast
tail of pancreas
tail of Spence
takeoff of a vessel

talar
talipes arcuatus
talipes calcaneovalgus
talipes calcaneovarus
talipes calcaneus
talipes cavovalgus
talipes cavus
talipes equinovalgus
talipes equinovarus
talipes equinus
talipes percavus
talipes planovalgus
talipes planus
talipes valgus
talipes varus
talocrural
talus
tampon
tamponade, cardiac
tangential cut
tangential scapular view
tangential view
tantalum ball
tarsal bone
tarsal-metatarsal joint
tarsal navicular
tarsometatarsal joint
tarsoptosis
tarsus
TAV (transcutaneous aorto-velography)
Tawara node
TBC (total body calcium)
Tc, Tc 99m (see *technetium)*
TE (echo time)
Teale amputation
tear, bucket-handle
TECA (technetium albumin) study

technetium (Tc, Tc 99m)
    Tc 99m albumin colloid
    Tc 99m albumin microspheres
    Tc 99m colloid
    Tc 99m DISIDA
    Tc 99m DMSA
    Tc 99m DTPA
    Tc 99m DTPA aerosol
    Tc 99m GHP
    Tc 99m HDP
    Tc 99m HIDA
    Tc 99m labeled stannous methyl-
      ene diphosphonate
    Tc 99m lidofenin
    Tc 99m MAA
    Tc 99m MDP
    Tc 99m medronate
    Tc 99m pentetic acid
    Tc 99m PIPIDA
    Tc 99m polyphosphate
    Tc 99m PYP (pyrophosphate)
    Tc 99m sodium pertechnetate
    Tc 99m sulfur colloid
technique
    background subtraction
    Dotter-Judkins
    double contrast
    Egan
    full bladder
    inversion-recovery
    in vivo
    Judkins
    low-dose film mammographic
    multiplanar
    partial saturation
    Seldinger
    Sones
    subtraction
    xenon 133
Teflon sling repair
tegmentum
telecurietherapy

Telepaque contrast medium
temporal lobe
temporomandibular joint (TMJ)
temporo-occipital
temporoparietal region
tendon
    Achilles
    hamstring
    heel
    insertion of
tennis elbow
tenting of diaphragm
tenting of hemidiaphragm
terminal ileum
Terry-Thomas sign
tertiary contraction
tesla (T)
test
    Rehfuss
    Rubin
testicle, testicular
tethered bowel sign
tetrad, Fallot
tetralogy of Fallot
texture, echo
thalamic
thalamus
thallium scan
thallium stress test
thallium 201 (Tl 201) imaging
thallium 201 scintigraphy
THE (transhepatic embolization)
thecal sac
thenar eminence
theory, quantum
TheraSeed implant
thermal equilibrium
thermal neutron
therminoluminescent dosimetry
thermistor plethysmography
thermogram, liquid crystal
thickened pleura

thickening
    gallbladder wall
    bowel wall
    inner table of frontal bone
    pleural
Thiemann disease
third portion of duodenum
Thixokon contrast medium
thoracic aorta
thoracic esophagus
thoracic outlet syndrome
thoracic scoliosis
thoracic spine
thoracic stomach
thoracic vertebrae
thoracentesis
thoraces or thoraxes (pl. of thorax)
thoracoabdominal aortic aneurysm
thoracolumbar injury
thoracolumbar scoliosis
thoracotomy tube
Thoratrast contrast medium
thorax, bony
thoraxes or thoraces (pl. of thorax)
thorium dioxide contrast medium
three-dimensional Fourier transform
    (3DFT) imaging
three-part fracture
thrombosed
thrombosis
    deep venous
    venous
thrombus
    intramural
    mural
through-and-through fracture
thumb, gamekeeper's
Thurston Holland sign
thymoma
thymus gland
thyroid cachexia
thyroid gland, retrosternal

thyroid nodule
thyroid radioiodine uptake
thyroiditis, Hashimoto
thyrotoxicosis
thyroxine radioisotope assay
    ($T_4$ RIA)
TI (inversion time)
tibial plafond fracture
tibial plateau
tibial plateau fracture
tibial tuberosity
tibia vara
tibiale posticum
tibiofibular joint; ligament
tibiotalar
tibiotarsal dislocation
Tillaux fracture
time
    acquisition
    echo (TE)
    esophageal transit
    gastric transit
    image acquisition
    interpulse
    inversion (TI)
    radionuclide esophageal dead
    emptying
    recovery
    relaxation
    repetition (TR)
    resolving
    scan
    small-bowel transit
    spin-lattice proton relaxation
    transit
time-density curve
tip of catheter
tissue
    adipose
    fatty
    fibrotic
    glandular

tissue *(cont.)*
  soft
  subcutaneous
tissue-equivalent phantom
tissue slice
titanium capsule
TLD (thermoluminescent dosimeter)
  rod
TMJ (temporomandibular joint)
  syndrome
toe, Morton
Tomocat contrast medium
tomogram, -graphy
tomographic cuts; slices
tomographic sections
tomographic study; view
tomography
  automated computerized axial
    (ACAT)
  computerized axial (CAT)
  dynamic computerized
  lateral
  quantitative computed (QCT)
  single photon emission computed
    (SPECT)
tomoscanner, Philips T-60
tongue of tissue
tonus
tophaceous gout
tophus (pl. tophi)
torsional stress
torsion fracture
torsion of fracture fragment
tortuosity
tortuous aorta
torus fracture
torus frontalis
torus palatinus
torus of the cortex
Toshiba TCT-80 CT scanner
total body calcium (TBC)
total body scanning

total condylar depression fracture
total hip replacement prosthesis
Towne projection; view
TR (repetition time)
TR/TE (repetition time/echo time)
trabecular bone
trabeculation
trace amount of radiopharma-
  ceutical
tracer
tracer accumulation, abnormal
tracer uptake, increased
trachea, tracheal
tracheobronchial foreign body
tracheobronchial tree
tracheoesophageal fistula
tract
  biliary
  digestive
  fistulous
  Flechsig
  GI (gastrointestinal)
  intestinal
  intrahepatic biliary
  lower
  respiratory
  sinus
  upper
  urinary
traction diverticulum
tragus
transaxillary lateral view
transbrachial
transcapitate fracture
transcatheter variceal embolization
transcervical femoral fracture
transcervical fracture
transcondylar fracture
transducer
  linear
  sector
transepiphyseal fracture

transfer, saturation
transfixing
transform
  fast Fourier
  Fourier
transhamate fracture
transhepatic embolization (THE)
transient
transit time
transitional vertebra
translucent
translumbar aortogram
transluminal angioplasty, percutaneous (PTA)
transluminal dilatation of superficial femoral artery
transmalleolar
transmutation
transpedicular decompression
transphyseal
transposition of great vessels
transradial styloid perilunate
  dislocation
transscaphoid perilunate dislocation
transthoracic
transudate
transtriquetral fracture-dislocation
transverse colon
transverse diameter
transverse facial fracture
transverse fracture
transverse maxillary fracture
transverse pelvic diameter
transverse plane
transverse presentation
transverse process
transverse section
trapezium bone
trapezoid bone of Henle
trapezoid bone of Lyser
trapping of radioisotope
trauma

traumatic arthrosis
traumatic dislocation
traumatic dissection
traumatism
traversing
tree
  biliary
  bronchial
  intrahepatic biliary
Treitz, ligament of
triangle
  Labbé
  Langenbeck
  Livingston
  Ward
triangular bone
triangular defect
triangular fibrocartilage complex
tricuspid valve
trifid stomach
triflanged nail
trigone
  Henke
  inguinal
  Pawlik
trimalleolar
trimalleolar fracture
triplane fracture
triquetral bone
triquetral fracture
triquetrolunate dislocation
triquetrum
triradiate cartilage
trochanter
  greater
  lesser
trochanteric
trochlea humeri
trochlea tali
trochlear notch
trochlear process
trophedema

trophic fracture
TR/TE (repetition time/echo time),
  short
TruCut biopsy needle
true conjugate
truncus arteriosus
TSPP rectilinear bone scan
T–tube cholangiogram
tubal insufflation
tubal pregnancy
tube
    Bardex
    Bilbao-Dotter
    chest
    Cope nephrostomy
    Dobbhoff
    drainage
    ET (endotracheal)
    fallopian
    large-caliber
    Miller-Abbott
    nephrostomy
    NG (nasogastric)
    orogastric
    Rehfuss
    T self-retaining drainage
    thoracotomy
    tracheostomy
tubercle
    adductor
    costal
    genial (of mandible) (not *genital*)
    Gerdy
    Ghon
tuberculosis
tuberculous osteomyelitis

tuberosity
    bicipital
    femoral
    greater
    iliac
    infraglenoid
    ischial
    radial
    ulnar
tuboplasty, balloon
tubular bone
tuft fracture
tumifying epiploitis
tumor
    Braun
    dermoid
    Ewing
    Klatzkin
    napkin ring
    neurogenic
    sessile
tumor blush
tumor mass
tumor recurrence
tunneling
tunnel view
turbinate bone
turcica, sella
two-dimensional (2-D) Fourier
    imaging
two-dimensional sector scan
two-part fracture
two-view chest x-ray
tympanic bone
tyropanoate sodium contrast
    medium

# U, u

UCG (ultrasonic cardiography)
ulcer
  active duodenal
  anastomotic
  anterior wall antral
  antral
  bear claw
  benign
  bleeding
  collar button-like
  Cruveilhier
  Curling
  Cushing
  duodenal
  esophageal
  gastric
  giant peptic
  greater curvature
  jejunal
  juxtapyloric
  lesser curvature
  linear
  malignant
  marginal
  minute bleeding
  mucosal
  necrotic
  patchy colonic
  penetrating
  peptic
  perforated
  perforating
  postbulbar duodenal
  postsurgical recurrent
  prepyloric gastric
  punched-out
  punctate
  pyloric channel

ulcer *(cont.)*
  rake
  recurrent
  Rokitansky-Cushing
  rose thorn
  round
  sea anemone
  secondary jejunal
  serpiginous
  stercoral
  stomal
  stress
  V-shaped
ulcer bed
ulcer crater
ulceration, marginal
ulcerative colitis
ulna
ulnar bone
ulnar hand
ulnar notch
ulnar styloid process
ulnar tubercle
ultrafast CT scan
ultrasonic cardiography (UCG)
ultrasonography (US)
ultrasound
  abdominal
  ADR
  B-mode
  Doppler
  endoscopic (EUS) Doppler
  fetal
  gallbladder
  gray-scale
  Hewlett-Packard
  high-resolution
  Hitachi

ultrasound *(cont.)*
    intrarectal
    Irex Exemplar
    real-time
    transthoracic
    VingMed
ultrasound probe
Ultravist contrast medium
UM 4 real-time sector scanner
umbilical catheter
umbilical hernia
umbilication
uncertainty principle
unciform bone
undisplaced fracture
unenhanced scan
ungual phalanx
ungual tuft
unguicular tuberosity
unicornuate uterus
unigravida
unilateral fracture
unilateral involvement
union of fracture fragments
unit
    EMI
    Hounsfield (on CT scan)
    rutherford (rd)
unit of measure
    becquerel (Bq)
    centimeter (cm)
    cubic centimeter (cc)
    deciliter (dl)
    femtoliter (fL)
    gauss (G)
    gram (gm)
    gray (Gy)
    international unit (IU)
    kilogram (kg)
    joule (J)
    kelvin (K)
    kiloelectron volt (keV or kev)

unit of measure *(cont.)*
    kilogram (kg)
    kilohertz (kHz)
    kilometer (km)
    liter (L)
    megacurie (MCi)
    megahertz (MHz)
    meter (m)
    microcurie
    milliampere (mA)
    millicurie (mCi)
    milliequivalent (mEq)
    milligram (mg)
    milliliter (ml)
    millimeter (mm)
    millimeter of mercury (mm Hg)
    millimole (mmol)
    milliroentgen (mR)
    milliunit (mU)
    rad
    roentgen (R)
    tesla (T)
unipara
unopacified
unresolved pneumonia
unstable fracture
ununited fracture
UPJ (ureteropelvic junction)
upper GI (gastrointestinal) series
upper lung field
upper mantle radiotherapy
upper thoracic esophagus
upright film; view
uptake
    diffuse
    heterogeneous
    iodine 131 metaiodobenzyl-
        guanidine
    radioiodine
    uniform
upward and backward dislocation
urachus

ureter
ureteral dilatation
ureterectasis
ureterocele
ureteropelvic junction (UPJ)
urethra, angle of inclination of
urethrogram, retrograde
urethrovesical angle
urinary tract
urogenital diaphragm
urogram, excretory
Urografin contrast medium
urokinase protocol
Urovist Cysto contrast medium
Urovist Meglumine contrast
   medium
Urovist Sodium contrast medium

US (ultrasonography) study
uterine fibroid
uterine neck
uterocervical
uterography
uteropelvic
uterosalpingography
uterotubography
uterovesical
uterus
   bicornis
   biforate
   bicornuate
   fibroid
   gravid
   unicornuate
uvula

# V, v

V-shaped fracture
vacuum cleft
vagina, vaginal
vaginogram
valgus carrying angle
valgus fracture, impacted
valgus, talipes
vallecula cerebelli
Valsalva maneuver
Valsalva, sinus of
valve
   Bauhin
   bicuspid
   Heister
   ileocecal
   mitral
   pyloric
   semilunar
   sigmoid

valve *(cont.)*
   tricuspid
   Vieussens
valve attenuation
valvulae conniventes
Vance dilator
Van de Graaff generator
Vaquez disease
variant
varices, esophageal
varioliform gastritis
varix (pl. varices)
varum, genu
varus deformity
varus, talipes
Vascoray contrast medium
vascular insult
vascular markings
vascular ring

vascularity
vasculature
Vater
  ampulla of
  papilla of
Vater diverticulum
VCUG (voiding cystourethrogram)
vein, azygos
velopharyngeal closure
velopharyngeal function
velopharyngeal structures
velum
Venable screw
vena cava
  inferior
  superior
venacavography
Venflon
venogram, isotope
venography
  adrenal
  iliac
  intraosseous
venous channel, deep
venous lake
venous scan
venous thrombosis
ventilation-perfusion (VQ) scan
ventilation, uneven
ventral hernia
ventricle, Verga
ventricle (of brain; heart; larynx)
ventricular ejection fraction
ventricular failure
ventricular system
ventriculocisternostomy
ventriculogram, radionuclide (RNV)
ventriculography, bubble
ventriculus cordis
Verga ventricle
vermicular appendage
vermiform appendix

vermiform process
vertebra, vertebrae
  cervical
  lumbar
  sacral
  thoracic
vertebral body
vertebral body endplate
vertebral stripe
vertebra plana fracture
vertebrocostal rib
vertebrophrenic angle
vertebrosternal rib
vertex presentation
vertical fracture
vertical plane
vertical shear fracture
vesical (adj.)
vesicle
  graafian
  malpighian
vesicula (pl. vesiculae)
vesicular
vesicoureterogram
vesicourethral angle
vesicovaginal fistula
vessel, vessels
  collateral
  great
  heart and great
  runoff
viable, viability
videofluoroscopy
videoradiography
Vieussens valve
view or projection (x-ray)
  abdominal
  afferent
  AP (anteroposterior)
  AP supine
  apical
  apical lordotic

view or projection *(cont.)*
   Arcelin
   axial sesamoid
   axillary
   baseline
   Beath
   Boehler calcaneal
   Boehler lumbosacral
   Breuerton
   Bucky
   Caldwell
   carpal tunnel
   Carter-Rowe
   Chamberlain-Towne
   Chausse
   cine
   coalition
   comparison
   coned
   coned-down
   coronal
   craniocaudad, craniocaudal
   cross-table lateral
   decubitus
   dens (cervical spine)
   dorsoplantar
   Dunlop-Shands
   efferent
   en face
   erect
   expiration
   Ferguson
   first-pass
   flexion
   fluoroscopic
   follow-through
   frogleg
   frogleg lateral
   frontal
   gated
   Granger
   Harris

view or projection *(cont.)*
   Harris-Beath
   heavily penetrated
   Hughston
   infrapatellar
   inspiration
   intraoperative
   inversion ankle stress
   Jones
   Jude pelvic
   LAO (left anterior oblique)
   LAO-cranial
   lateral
   lateral decubitus
   lateral oblique
   Law
   limited
   lordotic
   Low-Beers
   Mayer
   mediolateral
   mediolateral oblique
   mortise
   nonstanding lateral oblique
   notch
   oblique
   odontoid
   open-mouth odontoid
   optimally positioned
   overhead
   overhead oblique
   Owen
   PA (posteroanterior)
   plantar axial
   portable
   postevacuation
   preliminary
   prone
   push-pull ankle stress
   push-pull hip
   RAO (right anterior oblique)
   RAO-caudal

view or projection *(cont.)*
   recumbent
   Schüller
   scout
   sitting-up
   ski-jump
   skyline
   spider
   spot
   standing dorsoplantar
   standing lateral
   standing weightbearing
   Stenver
   stereoscopic
   submental vertex
   submentovertex
   sunrise
   sunset
   supine
   supine full
   swimmer's
   tangential scapular
   tomographic
   Towne
   transaxillary lateral
   transcranial lateral
   transscapular
   true lateral
   tunnel
   upright
   von Rosen
   Waters
   weeping willow

view or projection *(cont.)*
   weightbearing dorsoplantar
   White leg-length
viral pneumonia
Virchow psammoma
viscera (pl. of viscus)
visceral pleura
Vistec x-ray detectable sponge
visualization
   optimal
   poor
   suboptimal
vitelline duct
Vladimiroff-Mikulicz amputation
vocal cord
void (verb)
voiding cystourethrogram (VCUG)
voiding sequence
volar angulation
volar capsule
Volkmann deformity
Volkmann disease
Volkmann ischemic contracture
Volkmann subluxation
volume element (voxel)
volume loss
volvulus, cecal
vomer bone
von Gierke disease
von Recklinghausen disease
voxel (volume element)
VQ or V/Q (ventilation-perfusion)
   scan (Q means "quotient")

# W, w

W-shaped pouch
wagon wheel fracture
Wagstaffe fracture
Walcher position
Waldenström disease
wall
  bladder
  bowel
  intestinal
  luminal
  stomach
wall filter
wash-in phase
washout phase
water bath
water path
water range
water-soluble contrast agent
waterfall stomach
Waters projection; view
wave
  primary peristaltic
  secondary
  tertiary
wavelength, de Broglie
wedge compression fracture
wedge fracture
wedge, mediastinal
wedge-shaped mass
wedge-shaped vertebra
wedging deformity
weeping willow view
Wegner disease
weightbearing
weight, estimated fetal
Weitbrecht ligament

well-inflated lung
wet reading of x-ray film
whettle bone
White leg-length view
white-out of lungs
white matter infarct
Wiberg classification of patellar
  types
wide-mouth sac
widening of interpedicular distance
widespread involvement
wide window setting
Willis, circle of
willow fracture
Wilson cloud chamber
window, bone
wing, iliac
wing of ilium
Winslow, foramen of
wire
  guide
  monitoring
wire suture
Wirsung duct
womb
workup (n.), work up (v.)
wound
  closed
  exit
  gunshot
  open
  puncture
  stab
woven bone
wristdrop
wry neck (torticollis)

# X, x

X, Y, and Z coordinates for target
    lesion
xanthogranulomatous cholecystitis
xanthomatosis of long bones with
    spontaneous fracture
xenon 133 (Xe 133) radioisotope
xenon 133 ventriculography
xeromammogram
xeromammography
xeroradiogram
xerostomia
XIP (x-ray in plaster)
xiphisternal region
xiphoid angle

xiphoid area
xiphoid bone
xiphoid cartilage
xiphoid process
XOP (x-ray out of plaster)
x-ray
    baseline chest
    portable
x-ray film jacket
x-ray in plaster (XIP)
x-ray out of plaster (XOP)
x-ray tray, Bucky
x-ray view (see *view)*
Xylocaine

# Y, y

Y fracture
Y-T fracture

yoke
yokelike

# Z, z

Z-line of esophagus
Zang space
Zenker diverticulum
Zenker pouch
zero-field splitting
zeugmatography, Fourier trans-
    formation
Zickel nail
ZK44012 contrast medium
zonal gastritis

zone
    cross-sectional
    entry
    fracture
    lung
    portal
ZSC (zone of slow conduction)
zygapophyseal joint
zygoma
zygomatic arch; bone; process

# References

## Radiology

*American Journal of Roentgenology.* Baltimore: Williams and Wilkins Co., April and May 1989.

Hurley, Brenda J., and Richard J. Bagby, M.D. "Technical Advances in Radiology and Related Terminology Update," *Journal of the American Association for Medical Transcription,* Vol. 5, No. 3 (Fall 1986), 14-18.

*Pediatric Radiology,* multiple issues. New York: Springer International, 1989.

*Radiologic Clinics of North America,* multiple issues. Philadelphia: W. B. Saunders Co., 1989.

*Radiology,* multiple issues. Radiological Society of North America, Inc., 1988-1989.

Ravin, Carl E., M.D., and Robert H. Jones, M.D. "Radiologic Techniques for Diagnosis of Surgical Disorders, in *Textbook of Surgery,* 13th ed.. Edited by David C. Sabiston, Jr., M.D., 1986. Philadelphia: W. B. Saunders Co., 1986.

Sloane, Sheila B. *A Word Book in Radiology.* Philadelphia: W. B. Saunders Co., 1988.

Sochurek, Howard. "Medicine's New Vision," *National Geographic,* Vol. 171, No. 1 (January 1987), 2-41.

*A SUM Plus Exercise in Radiology and Pathology Transcription.* Modesto, Ca.: Health Professions Institute, 1988.

*The SUM Program Radiology Transcription Unit.* Modesto, Ca.: Health Professions Institute, 1987.

## General

Billups, Norman F., and Shirley M. Billups. *American Drug Index.* 33rd ed. Philadelphia: J. B. Lippincott Co., 1989.

*Cardiology Words and Phrases: A Quick-Reference Guide.* Modesto, Ca.: Health Professions Institute, 1989.

*Dorland's Illustrated Medical Dictionary.* 27th ed. Philadelphia: W. B. Saunders Co., 1988.

*Drug Facts and Comparisons.* St. Louis: J. B. Lippincott Co., 1989.

*GI Words and Phrases: A Quick-Reference Guide.* Modesto, Ca.: Health Professions Institute, 1989.

Lorenzini, Jean A. *Medical Phrase Index.* 2nd ed. Oradell, N.J.: Medical Economics Co., 1989.

*Orthopedic Words and Phrases: A Quick-Reference Guide.* Modesto, Ca.: Health Professions Institute, 1988.

*Physicians' Desk Reference.* 43rd ed. Oradell, N.J.: Medical Economics Co., 1989.

Pyle, Vera. *Current Medical Terminology.* 2nd ed. Modesto, Ca.: Prima Vera Publications, 1988.

Roe-Hafer, Ann. *The Medical & Health Sciences Word Book.* 2nd ed. Boston: Houghton Mifflin Co., 1982.

*Stedman's Medical Dictionary.* 25th ed. Baltimore: Williams & Wilkins Co., 1990.

*Taber's Cyclopedic Medical Dictionary.* 16th ed. Philadelphia: F. A. Davis Co., 1989.

*Webster's Medical Desk Dictionary.* Springfield, Mass.: Merriam-Webster, Inc., Publishers, 1986.

## Style

*American Medical Association Manual of Style,* 8th ed. Cheryl Iverson (Chair) et al. Edited by William Hensyl. Baltimore: Williams & Wilkins Co., 1989.

*Chicago Manual of Style.* 13th ed. Chicago: The University of Chicago Press, 1982.

Fordney, Marilyn T., and Marcy O. Diehl. *Medical Transcription Guide: Do's and Don'ts.* Philadelphia: W. B. Saunders Co., 1990.

Tessier, Claudia, and Sally C. Pitman. *Style Guide for Medical Transcription.* Modesto, Ca.: American Association for Medical Transcription, 1985.

## English Dictionaries

*The American Heritage Dictionary.* 2nd ed. New York: Houghton Mifflin Co., 1983.

*The New Lexicon Webster's Dictionary of the English Language.* New York: Lexicon Publications, Inc., 1987.

*Oxford American Dictionary.* Compiled by Eugene Ehrlich et al. New York: Oxford University Press, 1980.

*The Random House Dictionary of the English Language.* 2nd ed., Unabridged. Edited by Flexner and Hauck. New York: Random House, 1987.

*Webster's Ninth New Collegiate Dictionary.* Springfield, Mass.: Merriam-Webster, Inc., Publishers, 1988.

*Webster's Third New International Dictionary of the English Language, Unabridged.* Springfield, Mass.: Merriam-Webster, Inc., 1981.